You Too Can be Free from Asthma

For asthma, preventing its attack is more beneficial than treating its symptoms after it already occurs.

By James Liu, MD, PhD

YOU TOO CAN BE FREE FROM ASTHMA. Copyright© by James Z. Liu. All rights reserved. Printed in the United States of America. No part of this book may be used or reproduced in any manner whatsoever without written permission except in the case of brief quotations for noncommercial purposes. For information, please contact Dr. James Liu, 111 McCoy Street, Milford, DE 19963, USA.

ISBN-13: 978-1480256637
ISBN-10: 1480256633

Publisher's Note: Neither the publisher nor the author are engaged in providing professional medical advice or service to the individual reader. The content, ideas, procedures, and suggestions in this book are not intended as a substitute for professional medical attention. For all matters regarding your health and management of your asthma, please consult a health care professional. Neither the publisher nor the author is liable or responsible for any loss or damage allegedly arising from any material in this book. The author and publisher are not responsible for your specific health needs that may require medical supervision, nor any adverse reactions to any procedures or information provided in this book.

AUTHOR'S DISCLOSURE

Dr. James Liu is the author of this book as well as the proud inventor of a unique AsthmaCare™ Kit, which provides a remarkably effective solution for the management of asthma. Many friends of Dr. James Liu used this unique product to control their asthma attacks effectively. This book contains direct quotes from testimonials of actual users who were very satisfied after using the AsthmaCare™ Kit. The author was as objective as possible in presenting the facts, experiences, ideas, processes, approaches and suggestions within this book for the maximum benefit of readers. These statements have not been reviewed by the US Food and Drug Administration or other regulatory agencies.

DEDICATION

This book is dedicated to:

The contributors of the book who have suffered from asthma for years and then were asthma free for many days by using the preventive methods contained in this book; and to the readers who have a high likelihood of receiving benefits from reading this book.

Contents

1. A Worrisome Life with Asthma 1
Asthma is a Cruel and Dangerous Disease 1
    Whom Does Asthma Affect? 2
    Toll from the Rise in Asthma Cases 3
Common Asthma Flare-up Symptoms 4
Symptoms of Asthma Vary by Person 4
    New Hope for People with Asthma 6
2. Asthma Triggers 9
    Viral Infections Can Trigger Asthma 10
    Airborne Allergens Trigger Asthma 11
    Other Factors That Can Trigger Asthma 13
3. How an Asthma Attack is Triggered 17
    Respiratory Viruses 17
    Allergens 18
    Exercise 19
4. How to Avoid or Remove Asthma Triggers 23
    Avoid Eating Foods That Seem to Trigger Asthma 23
    Avoid Pollen or Outdoor Mold 23
    Remove Indoor Mold 23

Reduce Smoke 23
Avoid Strong Odors 24
Turn on the Air Conditioning 24
Keeping a Steady, Slow Pace While Exercising 24
Take Cover in Cold Weather 24
Control Pet Dander 24
Eliminate Mites and Cockroaches 24
Use Man-made Fibers, Not Feathers 25
Remove Viruses from the Upper Airway 25
    Cleansing Cold Viruses Can Cure Colds in One Day 25
How to Reduce the Cold Duration by More Than Four Days 26
    Viruses – A Numbers Game 27
    Know the Risks of Catching a Cold Virus 29
    How to Start Nasal Cleansing Sooner 30
    Where to Get an AsthmaCare™ Kit 30
    How to Use AsthmaCare™ Kit 30
    A Most Complete Nasal Cleansing Procedure 31
    Removing Residual Liquid 32
    Maintenance after Each Use 32
    How to Use the AsthmaCare™ Oral Spray 33

5. Drugs to Treat Asthma 35
Different Types of Asthma Medication 36
Long-Term Control Asthma Medications 36
Quick-Relief Asthma Medications 37
Over-the-Counter Asthma Drugs 38

Manage Your Asthma with Medications 38

6. Alternative Approaches to Treat Asthma 41

Acupuncture 41

Breathing exercises 41

Herbal remedies 42

Inspiration muscle training 43

Massage and chiropractic treatment 43

Relaxation therapy 43

Vitamins and supplements 43

7. Asthma Prevention 47

Flu Vaccination 47

Allergy Shots 48

Using Antibodies to Reduce Eosinophilic Asthma Attack 48

New Anti-IgE Drug to Reduce Asthma Attacks 49

Anti-Interleukin 13 (IL-13) Antibody 49

A Combinational Therapy 50

8. Homeopathy for Treating Asthma 53

9. Treat and Prevent Asthma Using 2-in-1 Therapy 61

The Environmental Load is Heavy 61

The Unmet Need is Great 61

The 2-in-1 Therapy 61

10. Frequently Asked Questions about Asthma 65

Glossary 73

References 81

About the Author 91

1. A Worrisome Life with Asthma

Asthma is a Cruel and Dangerous Disease

Asthma is a chronic inflammatory disorder of the airways in which many cells and cellular elements play a role. The chronic inflammation is associated with airway hyper-responsiveness that leads to recurrent episodes of wheezing, breathlessness, chest tightness, and coughing, particularly at night or in the early morning. These events are usually associated with widespread, but variable, airflow obstruction within the lung that is often reversible either spontaneously or with treatment." This definition was given by Global Initiative for Asthma in 2008 as part of the Global Strategy for Asthma Management and Prevention (Bateman 2008). "

Anyone who has experienced a severe asthma attack, with its accompanying feelings of fear, panic, and helplessness, knows that this disease can be cruel and dangerous.

Before an attack, people with asthma often have symptoms of sneezing, drowsiness, restlessness, and/or irritability. There can also be a dry cough accompanied by a wheezing breathlessness. During an actual asthma attack, there is a sudden heaviness in the chest, especially at night, as well as a feeling of suffocation that leaves a person fighting for air to breathe.

Anxiety, perspiration, cold extremities and cyanosis are often present during an asthma attack. Wheezing becomes more pronounced and can be heard from a distance. The airway can become so obstructed during an attack that the chest is almost silent when a physician uses a stethoscope to listen to the lungs (auscultation). Physicians often find that inhalation is short and high pitched while exhalation is prolonged and labored. On auscultation, a physician will hear many abnormal sounds inside the chest. If the asthma attack lasts for many hours with paroxysms (spasms), it becomes asthmaticus, or a severe asthmatic attack. In this state, the patient must be admitted to a hospital for oxygen and other supportive treatments.

While asthma is a chronic condition that can flare up at any time, asthma symptoms tend to worsen late at night. Possible reasons for this worsening at night include:

1) **The body's internal clock.** The body produces certain substances that protect against inflammation. Levels of these substances can be lower at night, which may contribute to a worsening of symptoms during the night.

2) **Sinus infections or postnasal drip due to allergens.** At night, there is a continual inhalation of allergens, such as dust mites or pet dander, without an opportunity to expel the allergens.

3) **Heartburn.** Stomach acid backing up into the esophagus or throat causes heartburn, which is often a sign of gastroesophageal reflux disease (GERD). When suffering from a GERD attack, lying down can make heartburn worse, aggravating asthma symptoms. If asthma symptoms tend to worsen at night, do not eat too close to bedtime, and ask a healthcare provider about GERD. Treating GERD may help to improve asthma symptoms in people who have both conditions.

Cessation of an asthma attack can be spontaneous or due to medication. As the bronchial spasms lessen, breathing eases and coughing is more productive, bringing out thick and sticky sputum.

Complications from asthma attacks also vary significantly. These include respiratory fatigue, pneumothorax (a collapsed lung), atelectasis (the collapse of part or all of a lung), pneumomediastinum (air in the mediastinum, which is the mass of tissues separating the two pleural sacs of the lung), and side effects from the medications used. Death can even occur, if the attack is severe enough or left untreated too long.

Whom Does Asthma Affect?

How common is asthma? According to the World Health organization (WHO), 300 million people worldwide have asthma; this is about equal to the entire population of the Unites States. In the

US alone, 25.7 million Americans suffer from asthma. Each year, asthma is responsible for roughly half a million hospital stays, one quarter of all emergency room visits, and 4,000 deaths.

For example, in 2003, asthma prevalence in the State of Delaware equaled the national prevalence, as did its asthma-related hospital discharge rate. According to the Delaware Behavioral Risk Factor Survey (Report Details Asthma Prevalence and Burden in Delaware, August 2005), 11.7% of adults in Delaware reported having asthma at some time during their lives, and 7.5% of adults currently have the disease.

Asthma appears to be slightly more prevalent among young people. As reported in the 2003 Delaware Youth Risk Behavior Survey, about 19% of high school students reported having been diagnosed with asthma; and 6.5% said they had an asthma attack in the past 12 months.

For some people, asthma is intermittent and well controlled, while for others, it is persistent and uncontrolled. Comparatively, asthma is less common in adults than in children and adolescents; among children, asthma is the most common chronic ailment. As stated in the Delaware Asthma Burden report, children under age 4 are more than twice as likely to be hospitalized with asthma as any other age group and about four times as likely as adults to have an asthma-related hospitalization. The report estimates there are about 3,000 asthma-related hospitalizations of children per year.

Asthma also affects productivity and quality of life. About 23% of adults with asthma were unable to work or carry out daily activities for one or more days during the past month.

Toll from the Rise in Asthma Cases

Asthma is on the rise; the incidence of asthma in the U.S. has nearly doubled in the last 15 years across all age, sex, and ethnic groups. An estimated 25.7 million Americans had asthma in 2010 (Akinbami 2012). These numbers are causing considerable concern and confusion for public health experts as well as doctors. Although the exact reason for this increase is unknown, some medical researchers believe that growing exposure to certain chemicals is responsible for the rise. While there is no cure for asthma, there has been significant progress in the management of this chronic condition.

However, this need for ongoing management of asthma can have enormous economic ramifications. In Delaware only, asthma-related Medicaid charges totaled $13.9 million in 2003; the cost of asthma medications alone was $9.7 million, up from $4.4 million in 2000. Total statewide charges for asthma treatment and medications could be as high as $25 to $30 million a year (Report Details Asthma Prevalence and Burden in Delaware, August 2005).

Common Asthma Flare-up Symptoms

Unfortunately, asthma flare-ups can occur any time at work, at home, or at play. Not all asthma flare-ups are the same, as each person has their own unique set of symptoms during a flare-up. The most common asthma symptoms are:

1) Uncontrollable coughing, especially at night
2) Wheezing, or a high-pitched whistling sound when exhaling
3) Shortness of breath
4) Pain and/or pressure in the chest
5) Tightened neck and chest muscles
6) Trouble speaking
7) Anxiety or panic
8) Pale, clammy face due to lack of oxygen
9) Blue lips or fingernails due to lack of oxygen

Symptoms of Asthma Vary by Person

Not all people with asthma experience the same symptoms in the same way during each flare-up. They may not have all of these symptoms, or they may have different symptoms at different times. Their asthma symptoms may also vary from one asthma attack to the next, being mild during one occurrence and then severe during the next one.

In infants and children, a diagnosis of wheezy bronchitis, asthmatic bronchitis, or reactive airway disease (RAD) is not the same as a diagnosis of asthma, although these conditions can eventually lead to asthma. Fortunately, many asthmatic children grow out of the condition and, by adulthood, no longer have asthma attacks.

Most people with asthma can have happy and active lives, sometimes with restrictions, such as limiting the amount of exposure to cold air or the vigorousness of exercise. Some people with asthma may have asthma-free days for extended periods before a flare-up happens. When this period is interrupted by more frequent and/or severe bouts of asthma symptoms, these bouts are called asthma attacks or flare-ups. Some people might have asthma symptoms every day while other people may only have asthma after infection by cold viruses, during the spring allergy season, or during exercise.

Mild asthma attacks are more common. Usually, the partially closed airways re-open within a few minutes to a few hours. Severe flare-ups are less common, but last much longer and usually require immediate medical help. It is important to recognize and treat any asthma, even mild asthma symptoms, to help prevent severe flare-ups and keep asthma under control.

Although asthma has many triggers, there are four basic types categorized by the specific asthma-triggering agent. This is why it is a good idea for those with asthma to know what type they have in order to avoid the specific triggering agent. The four types are:

1) **Allergic asthma (extrinsic/atopic).** This type of asthma usually starts in childhood. Most children who develop allergic asthma also had bouts of eczema before the onset of the asthma. Most adults who develop asthma at age 35 years or less fall into this category as well. It is believed that genetic factors play a significant role in the development of allergic asthma. In this type of asthma, the allergen causes an excessive production of immunoglobulin E (IgE).

2) **Infective asthma.** This type of asthma is caused by, or at least associated with, an upper respiratory tract or bronchial infection from exposure to cold or flu viruses.

3) **Psychological asthma.** This type is closely related to anxiety, emotional stress, etc., and is often considered the sole cause of some asthma attacks. It is still not certain whether it is the sole cause or is only a precipitating factor.

4) **Occupational asthma.** This can occur in certain industries where exposure to certain substances such as chemicals, metallic dusts (such as platinum salts), biological detergents, and flour and dust from grains can cause asthma attacks.

Different types of asthma require different therapies. Infective asthma and allergy-related asthma are the most common types, but neither one can be preemptively treated in a conventional manner. Antiviral drugs that treat colds or the flu do not exist and, unless the specific allergen is known and can be avoided, allergy-related asthma cannot be prevented, either. So, are there viable treatment options for people with asthma?

Yes, there is! There is a new way to manage asthma in order to live a normal or near-normal life by controlling asthma flare-ups before they become attacks.

New Hope for People with Asthma

Many people have enjoyed numerous asthma-free days after using a very simple method to rid themselves of their asthma triggers. For people who have suffered too much from asthma, it is time to find a safe and effective method to have as many asthma-free days as possible. Any asthma-free day is priceless. If more asthma-free days are achievable, then why not get them! The following chapters will show the what, why, and how of obtaining asthma-free days.

1. A Worrisome Life with Asthma   7

8   You Too Can be Free from Asthma

2. Asthma Triggers

Each asthma attack has its unique precondition. A number of factors, called asthma triggers, generate this precondition. The most common asthma triggers are cold viruses, various allergens, animal dander, air pollution, smoke, mold, cold air, coughing, stress, exercise, or acid reflux.

Asthma is classified as either extrinsic asthma or intrinsic asthma. Extrinsic asthma is triggered by known or unknown external pathogens, such as viruses or allergens. Intrinsic asthma refers to those cases where no environmental factors are present and skin allergy tests are negative.

Two factors largely determine whether an asthma attack will occur. One is an internal factor, which is the reactive airway of patients with asthma and the other is an external factor, which is the environmental asthma trigger. Asthma flare-ups vary from person to person; however, one thing is consistent for all people with asthma. When the airway is exposed to enough asthma triggers for a long enough period, it becomes inflamed, causing it to narrow and fill with mucus.

For people with asthma, it is important for them to understand the many possible asthma triggers. Once the specific triggers are identified, people with asthma can take an active role in controlling their asthma and reducing the frequency of asthma attacks by decreasing exposure to these triggers, or by performing the right procedures to remove the inhaled triggers. In addition, being aware of environmental triggers, such as certain foods or high pollen counts, can help those with asthma to avoid them altogether, which can significantly reduce the frequency or severity of asthma attacks. If environmental pollution is the cause of asthma, it is important to stay indoors during periods of heavy pollen pollution. So what are the most common asthma triggers?

Viral Infections Can Trigger Asthma

Many respiratory viral infections can trigger asthma attacks. Numerous scientific studies demonstrate that infections from common respiratory viruses, such as cold viruses, influenza viruses, parainfluenza viruses, or respiratory syncytial virus (RSV), can trigger asthma attacks.

Many medical researchers have observed that the majority of asthma exacerbations are associated with respiratory tract viral infections. Respiratory viruses infect the bronchial epithelial cells on the surface of the airway, resulting in epithelial activation and increased recruitment and activation of white blood cells, in the form of neutrophils. In addition, viruses such as influenza and RSV can cause extensive epithelial necrosis (cell death) that is enhanced by the neutrophils. Necrosis of epithelial cells and white blood cells leads to the release of intracellular contents that may cause inflammatory reaction and trigger asthma attacks.

1) There is evidence that viral infections during early childhood can cause the immune system to increase the subsequent risk of asthma and allergen sensitization. One example is severe infection from RSV. Why does this happen? Medical researchers believe viral infections can increase the risk of asthma attack: Viral infections can increase airway responsiveness. The airway's reaction towards foreign substances becomes oversensitive, and the responsive reaction is at its maximal speed and intensity. That is why asthma flare-ups are so sudden and so severe.

2) Viral infections can alter normal immunity, which can prevent the immune system from sending the right signals to fight against a virus infection. Any inhaled viruses could then cause the inflammation necessary to trigger an asthma attack.

3) Viral infections can alter small airway geometry. After a viral respiratory tract infection, the airway wall becomes thick (edema), the lumen (space of the tubing airway) becomes narrow and plugged, the mucus secretions become excessive, and damaged airway cells leave their debris to cause further blockage in the airway. All of these changes contribute to the development of shortness of breath and asthma flare-ups.

4) Viral infections can cause increased airway inflammation. Both nonspecific and specific immune responses become more active. Airway epithelial cells, endothelial cells, macrophages, monocytes, granulocytes are on high alert status. There are also extremely active T-cell responses to the viral infection, a hyperactive combination of antigen-independent and antigen-specific responses, and over-strong interactions with the preexisting airway inflammation.

A physician can provide care when a person with asthma develops a cold or infection. It is also a good idea to get an annual flu shot, and, most importantly, try to stay healthy by eating right, exercising, and avoiding others who are suffering from a cold or the flu.

Airborne Allergens Trigger Asthma

Airborne allergies are common asthma triggers. Eighty percent of people with asthma have allergies to airborne substances such as tree, grass, weed, pollens, mold, animal dander, dust mites, and cockroach particles. In one study, children who had high levels of cockroach droppings in their homes were four times more likely to have childhood asthma than children whose homes had low levels. Asthma exacerbation after dust exposure is usually due to a dust mite allergy.

During the allergy season, pollen counts are high. Inhaling airborne pollens makes it easy to reach the threshold, or critical point, that triggers an asthma flare-up. This is considered a high-risk period and special attention should be paid for prevention and treatment of asthma.

Every year, the Asthmas and Allergy Foundation of America (AAFA) names the top 10 worst cities for asthma in the United States. Twelve factors are used to create the list, including air pollution, pollen, asthma rates, use of "rescue inhalers," and poverty. People with asthma who live in one of these cities should take special precautions to protect themselves. In order, the worst cities for 2012 as listed on www.asthmacapitals.com were:

1. **Memphis, Tennessee.** Memphis topped the 2012 list with high asthma death rates, weak smoking restrictions, poor air quality, and high poverty rates.

2. **New Haven, Connecticut.** Asthma cases have been on the rise in New Haven, where pollution and pollen are common triggers and smoking is still allowed in public places. Nurses and other health care providers are making home visits to help reduce asthma attacks among children.

3. **Knoxville, Tennessee.** Knoxville remains near the top of the worst city rankings. It has been one of the worst asthma cities year after year, like many other cities across the South and Southwest. Even though Knoxville has a better-than-average number of allergy specialists to treat people with asthma, the city is still vexed by poor air quality, incomplete smoke-free laws, and above-average use of asthma rescue medications.

4. **Pittsburgh, Pennsylvania.** This former steel town still has the worst air pollution in the country. With poor air quality, high pollen, and a lack of strict smoking bans, Pittsburgh has a very high rate of asthma.

5. **Chattanooga, Tennessee.** Poor air quality, pollen, and poverty help keep Chattanooga near the top of the worst asthma cities list. Like many Southern cities, Chattanooga lags behind in creating smoke-free laws that help clear the air of secondhand smoke in public places.

6. **Hartford, Connecticut.** This small state capital has a growing asthma problem, according to the AAFA. It jumped from No. 40 to No. 6 in just one year. High pollen counts and a lack of strict smoking bans contribute to this poor rating, making life more difficult for people with asthma.

7. **St. Louis, Missouri.** High pollen counts, a high poverty rate, and the lack of a widespread smoking ban in public places add up to big asthma issues here, according to the AAFA. Yet, life for people with asthma may have gotten a little better. St. Louis has improved in the rankings since it was named the worst city for people with asthma in 2009.

8. **Oklahoma City, Oklahoma.** Despite the efforts of the Oklahoma Asthma Initiative, the city moved up four spots to No. 8. The initiative's focus is to raise awareness about

asthma, especially among children, their parents, and teachers. Children are more likely to have asthma than adults are; as a result, asthma is the most common health reason for repeated absences from school.

9. **McAllen, Texas.** In the border town of McAllen, Texas, the problem is access to effective asthma treatments. Compared to other cities, more people in McAllen lack insurance and need "rescue" medications for asthma that is not well controlled. High poverty is linked to higher rates of asthma and McAllen is one of the poorest cities in the country.

10. **Allentown, Pennsylvania.** The city itself is not a pretty picture for people with asthma. Poor air quality, weak smoking bans in public places, and a high number of people with asthma pushed Allentown into the top 10 worst asthma capitals.

More and more studies show that allergies and asthma often occur together. The same substances that trigger allergy symptoms may also cause asthma symptoms, such as shortness of breath, wheezing and chest tightness. This is called allergic asthma or allergy-induced asthma.

How are allergies and asthma related? An allergic response occurs when antibodies generated by the immune system mistakenly treat a harmless substance as a dangerous invader. In an attempt to protect the body from the "harmful" substance, antibodies wrongly attack the substance (allergen). The chemicals released by the immune system lead to allergy symptoms, such as nasal congestion, runny nose, itchy eyes or skin reactions. For many people, this same reaction also affects the lungs and airways, leading to asthma symptoms.

Other Factors That Can Trigger Asthma

Besides viruses and allergens, many other factors contribute to the onset of an asthma attack:

1. Food allergies can trigger mild to severe asthma. The most common food allergens are eggs, cow's milk, peanuts, soy, wheat, fish, shrimp and other shellfish, salads and some

fresh fruits. Food preservatives can also trigger asthma. Sulfite additives, such as sodium bisulfite, potassium bisulfite, sodium metabisulfite, potassium metabisulfite, and sodium sulfite, are commonly used in food processing or preparation. They can trigger asthma in those people who are sensitive.

2. Indoor mold can also trigger an asthma attack if the spores are breathed in. Molds can hide anywhere in the house, especially in areas with high humidity because the added moisture encourages the mold to grow.

3. Smoking and special odors can cause or aggravate asthma symptoms. Smoking directly can trigger an asthma flare-up as can second-hand smoke from cigarettes, pipes, or even a stove. Perfumes, paints, hair spray, and powders can also exaggerate asthma symptoms. In addition, these scents and odors often linger in the house long after the source has departed.

4. Physical exercise is another trigger for asthma flare-ups. Too much exercise and/or exercising outdoors in the cold and dry air can exacerbate asthma flare-ups. Always consult a doctor before starting any exercise program. Aerobic exercise that repeatedly provokes an attack should be avoided and warming up prior to exercising is critical.

5. Breathing in cold air increases the risk of an asthma attack due to the hypersensitivity of the airway of people with asthma. Care should be taken during the winter months and/or in higher elevations in order to avoid possible asthma flare-ups.

6. Pet dander is one of the leading causes of an asthma attack as it can easily spread throughout the home. Either a person with asthma's own pet or someone else's can trigger asthma.

7. Mites and cockroaches can trigger an asthma attack. Areas with uncontrolled populations of cockroaches generally have higher rates of asthma.

8. Natural fibers are also recognized asthma triggers. While feather and down pillows, quilts, and cushions may be

comfortable, they can make asthma attacks infinitely worse. Instead, use ones filled with synthetic fibers. Also, consider replacing curtains with blinds, and carpets with wood floors to help cut down on allergens.

9. Drugs. Some drugs are known to trigger an attack so these drugs should be avoided. For example, Aspirin, the commonly used painkiller, or beta-blockers commonly prescribed medications to treat heart conditions, high blood pressure, and migraine headache.

10. In adults, psychological stress due to excess worry and stress can trigger an asthma attack as can overexcitement or overstimulation in children.

11. Occupational exposure can instigate an asthma attack. In a working environment, many people are exposed to a variety of harmful substances, such as chemicals, paint fumes, and other airborne irritants. People can have asthma that is specific to their working environment, such as meat wrappers' asthma, bakers' asthma, and wood workers' asthma.

It is important to know that these triggers may act alone, or in conjunction with each other. Special attention should be paid to avoid these triggers or remove them altogether. Several chapters of this book will illustrate how to deal with these common asthma triggers.

3. How an Asthma Attack is Triggered

Respiratory Viruses

Respiratory viruses are well recognized as major triggers of asthma attacks in children and adults, resulting in frequent outpatients visits and hospitalizations. New molecular diagnostic methods are being used to learn the pathophysiological mechanisms of how asthma is triggered by viral infection.

Almost thirty years ago, the association between viral infections and the exacerbation of asthma in children was found using tissue cultures and serological methods of detecting viruses. Subsequently, other studies using similar methods reported comparable findings in both adults and children. However, respiratory viruses are difficult to detect by standard methods, and therefore, earlier studies may have underestimated the impact of viral infections on asthma-related wheezing.

Upon the development of highly sensitive laboratory methods, such as RT-PCR assays, researchers began investigating the relationship between viral infections and asthma severity. In a 1993 study of 138 adults with asthma, Dr. Nicholson and his associates collected nose and throat swabs and blood samples to compare with collections from other adults who had no asthma symptoms. Their study showed that 75 percent of cold viruses were associated with asthma attacks (Nicholson 1993).

Dr. Johnston and colleagues performed a similar study in nine- to eleven-year-old children in 1995. Viruses were detected in 80 percent of reported episodes of asthma, with the rhinovirus identified most often. They also reported that the seasonal patterns of upper respiratory tract infection correlated with hospital admissions for asthma, but the relationship was stronger for pediatric than for adult admissions (Johnson 195).

A study by Dr. Zhu and associates went further in answering why the rhinovirus infection triggers asthma attacks (Zhu 2009). It is well known in the medical community that nasal mucociliary clearance is a critical innate defense system responsible for clearing up invading pathogens, including bacteria and viruses. At the right amounts, mucus is beneficial, but too much mucus blocks the airways and can exacerbate disease symptoms. In their study, the researchers found that both major and minor groups of rhinovirus-induced mucus production in primary human epithelial cells and cell lines. This suggests that viral-induced mucus overproduction may contribute to virus-induced airway disease exacerbation, including asthma.

Certain clinical studies show that respiratory viruses are present in most patients hospitalized for either life-threatening asthma or acute nonlife-threatening asthma. Rhinovirus is the most common, but co-infection with other viruses may be important. Although patients with asthma are not more susceptible to upper respiratory tract rhinovirus infections than healthy people are, they do suffer from more severe consequences of lower respiratory tract inflammation. That leads to the question of why an asthma patient's internal system responds so differently to a viral infection.

Recent medical studies suggest that viruses inflame asthma attacks by additive or synergistic interactions with allergen exposure or with air pollution. A weakened antiviral immunity to the rhinovirus may lead to weakened viral clearance and consequently, prolonged symptoms. Respiratory viral infections cause asthmatic exacerbations by triggering recruitment of special immune cells (Th2-type cells) into the lungs.

If medication cannot inhibit a viral infection, there are other methods to help reduce viral asthma triggers. These methods are discussed in Chapter 4.

Allergens

Besides allergic related immunoglobulin E (IgE), the immune system produces immunoglobulin G (IgG) in response to common inhalant allergens. Increased serum titers of allergen-specific IgG, whether induced spontaneously or by allergen vaccination, have been implicated in protection against asthma. Scientists conducted further tests to verify the interference of topical IgG with the allergen-triggered eosinophilic airway inflammation that underlies asthma. They treated allergen-sensitized mice by intranasal instillation of specific IgG, followed by the specific allergen challenge. These animals were protected by adding anti-allergen IgG before they were given the allergen. The results provide a basis for topical immunotherapy of asthma by direct delivery of anti-allergen IgG to the airways (Sehra 2003). If both IgE and allergen are suppressed, asthma attacks should be reduced.

If asthma-specific IgG and/or IgE cannot be suppressed with traditional asthma medications, there are other methods available, which will be covered in Chapter 4.

Exercise

Exercise-induced asthma, or EIA, refers to the transient narrowing of the airways that follows vigorous exercise (Anderson 2000). The mechanism that causes EIA is thought to relate to the consequences of heating and humidifying large volumes of air during exercise. In 1978, airway cooling was first identified as an important stimulus for EIA; however, severe EIA also occurred when hot dry air was inhaled, and there was no abnormal cooling of the airways. In 1986, the thermal hypothesis proposed that cooling of the airways followed by rapid re-warming, caused vasoconstriction and reactive hyperemia (an increase in the quantity of blood) of the bronchial microcirculation. This, combined with edema of the airway wall, causes the airways to narrow after exercise, prompting an asthma attack (Anderson 2000).

Cooling and rapid re-warming of the airways occurs when cold air is inhaled during exercise, but these events are not always necessary for EIA to occur. Hyperpnoea (an increased depth of breathing when required to meet metabolic demand of body tissues) with cold dry air should be considered not only for its capacity to cool the airways but also for its potential to involve smaller airways in the humidifying process and, as a result, becoming dehydrated and hyperosmolar (electrolytes concentration is too high because airway lost too much water). The mechanism for EIA could be due to the dehydrating effects of respiratory water loss that leads to the release of inflammatory mediators. In another words, cell shrinkage could lead to the release of inflammatory mediators. Potentially, all airway cells, such as epithelial cells, mast cells, eosinophils, macrophages, and sensory nerve cells, are subject to cell volume loss after dehydration. The airways are narrowed by contraction of bronchial smooth muscles in response to the mediators and the effect will be amplified in the presence of airway edema.

As water is evaporated from the airway surface, the solution in the airway becomes hyperosmolar (electrolytes abnormally higher) and provides an osmotic stimulus for water to move from any cell nearby, resulting in cell volume loss. In addition, patients with asthma have a slower rate of transfer of water to the airway surface because of airway inflammation. The airway-surface-liquid volume is normally 1 milliliter (mL). It is easy to lose water from cells, but not as easy to replace. Cell shrinkage is the key event in the release of inflammatory mediators that cause airway smooth muscles to contract and the airways of people with asthma to narrow.

3. How an Asthma Attack is Triggered

4. How to Avoid or Remove Asthma Triggers

Once asthma triggers are known, people with asthma are able to take whatever possible approaches they can to avoid or remove them. This chapter explains some safe methods that can be used.

Avoid Eating Foods That Seem to Trigger Asthma

Sensitivity to certain foods and drinks, like shrimp, dried fruit, processed potatoes, beer, or wine, can aggravate asthma symptoms. Speak with a physician about the best ways to change food habits to avoid potential asthma attacks. If a person with asthma has a food allergy, those foods should be avoided completely.

Avoid Pollen or Outdoor Mold

During allergy season, consider staying inside from midday through the afternoon, when pollen counts are at their peak. Close all doors and windows to keep out airborne pollens and molds that may trigger an asthma attack. Ask a physician if adjusting asthma treatment during these high-risk periods would be beneficial.

Remove Indoor Mold

Fix leaky faucets and pipes. Use bleach to clean any mold lingering on shower curtains and surfaces. However, care should be taken as bleach can trigger an asthma attack. Always wear a mask or ask someone else to clean the mold. Added moisture encourages mold growth; using a dehumidifier can thwart mold growth.

Reduce Smoke

Smoke from cigarettes, pipes, or even a stove may irritate asthma symptoms. Smoking also lowers immunity, making people with asthma more susceptible to viral infections that increase inflammation, which can lead to attacks that are more frequent. The best course of action is to quit smoking.

Avoid Strong Odors

Special perfumes, paints, and powders have strong odors that often linger in the house long after the source has departed. Avoid using them as much as possible.

Turn on the Air Conditioning

If airborne pollens and molds trigger asthma attacks, closing the windows and using the air conditioner can lessen exposure because the air conditioner filters out a large amount of these common allergens.

Keeping a Steady, Slow Pace While Exercising

By warming up gradually before exercising allows the airway to better tolerate cold or dry air. When exercising outside during the colder months, keep a slow, steady pace to avoid large influxes of cold and/or dry air. If asthma symptoms act up, take a break and treat the symptoms as directed by a physician. Of course, always take any recommended medications as prescribed, as well as consult a physician before starting any exercise program.

Take Cover in Cold Weather

Covering the nose and mouth with a scarf on cold or windy days helps to avoid asthma symptoms.

Control Pet Dander

Pets are well-known asthma triggers. Pet dander easily spreads throughout the home; therefore, keeping pets clean and away from the bedroom helps immensely in cutting down on exposure. In addition, furniture should be covered, carpets should be periodically cleaned, and even stuffed toys should be washed periodically.

Eliminate Mites and Cockroaches

To reduce exposure to dust mites, cover mattresses and box springs with dust-proof covers, wash all bedding in hot water (at least 130° F) once a week, and vacuum once a week. To avoid cockroaches, use traps and avoid leaving food out.

Use Man-made Fibers, Not Feathers

While feather and down pillows, quilts, and cushions may be comfortable and warm, they may also cause severe asthma flare-ups. Instead, use ones filled with synthetic fibers. Also, consider replacing curtains with blinds, and carpets with wood floors.

Remove Viruses from the Upper Airway

The upper airway is notorious for harboring cold and other respiratory viruses. The upper airway is the portion of the respiratory tract that extends from the nostrils or mouth through the larynx. The major part of the upper airway is the nasal cavity, but it also contains parts of the pharynx.

Normal breathing utilizes parts of the upper and lower airways. The lower airway stretches from the inferior end of the larynx to the ends of the terminal bronchioles; the lungs are the primary organ of the lower airway. Physicians often refer to asthma as "one airway, one disease". This is because, even though the airway is broken into two distinct areas, they are both equally involved in asthma flare-ups. A narrowing of the bronchioles, which are small-branched airways in the lungs, causes the breathlessness and wheezing during an asthma attack, while the triggers that cause an attack usually reside in the upper airway.

Regularly cleansing the upper airway of existing viruses helps to disarm these asthma triggers. However, is this even possible?

Cleansing Cold Viruses Can Cure Colds in One Day

Dr. James Liu, the author of this book, has firsthand experience in cleansing out cold viruses from his nasal cavity:

> *For the last five years, I rarely had the common cold as I regularly perform nasal cleanse during the cold months. One exception was October 17, 2010 when I had a long day driving from Boston MA to Downingtown PA after meeting many tradeshow participants. I did not perform a nasal cleanse because I was too tired. Clearly, I had cold symptoms on October 18, 2010 when I was working in my office. Immediately, I performed a complete nasal cleanse with the NasalCare® Nasal*

> Cleanse Kit every 4 hours on that day. My cold symptoms were all gone the next day. My son had the same experience when he had a cold in April 2011. He recovered the next day after performing a number of nasal cleanses. My office manager got the same result when she performed nasal cleanse 4 times on September 7, 2012, and her common old symptoms all disappeared the next day. Without effectively cleansing out these cold viruses, we cannot cure our colds in just one day.

How to Reduce the Cold Duration by More Than Four Days

As reported in a published clinical study (Ao 2011), medical researchers determined that cold and/or flu viruses could be removed by performing nasal irrigation three times a day. During a baseline visit on Day 1, the patients who presented with either a cold or the flu had not performed nasal irrigation yet. Their nasal secretions tested positive for the influenza virus. After performing nasal irrigation three times a day for three days, all patients, who had previously tested positive for the influenza virus, now became virus negative at their Day 4 office visit. The cold and/or flu symptoms of these patients had also disappeared. During the next office visit on day 8, all these patients were tested again and no viruses were detected.

The true efficacy of nasal cleanses would be much clearer if the patients could be tested every day to determine levels of virus infection. However, it is not practicable to conduct daily "best tests" in real life. Because the patients could not come to the clinic every day to test for viruses in their nasal secretions, there was a chance that these viruses were cleansed out even before the Day 4 office visit.

Many people may wonder if effectively removing the viruses that cause colds and/or the flu could result in a quicker recovery. In a word, yes. As reported by these medical researchers, the majority of patients with colds or the flu who used the NasalCare® Cleanse Kit to treat their viral infection reduced the severity of their cold symptoms in just one day after performing an effective nasal cleansing under a physician's direction. After two days of treatment with the NasalCare® Cleanse System three times a day, their cold symptoms were significantly less severe than those patients in the comparison group who did not use the kit, and they recovered much faster. On an average basis, their cold duration was reduced by 4.5 days, as compared to the patients who did not perform a nasal cleanse.

Although this was not an asthma study, the effectiveness of the NasalCare® Nasal Cleanse System in removing cold viruses can be used as an example for asthma patients as to how performing a nasal cleanse can get rid of these cold viruses from the nasal cavity and possibly reduce the frequency and/or severity of asthma attacks.

Many people with asthma have used the NasalCare® Nasal Cleanse System to reduce their asthma flare-ups with great success:

"I love my NasalCare! I use it almost every day. I ran out of your mix packets a few months ago. I had to buy the store brand, and they are not as good. It really helps me a lot. I tell everyone about it. I still have flare-ups in the fall and spring, but nothing like I had before. When it gets bad, I use it every day, sometimes twice a day. I would love some more of your packets.' *Suzanne K., Tennessee.*

"I have allergies & asthma. Since I have been using NasalCare I have noticed such a relief in my symptoms. It is nice to be able to breathe clearly again. I really love it; so easy to use and it works!" *Karen M., North Carolina*

Viruses – A Numbers Game

So, how many viruses need to be removed from the nose in order to feel relief from a cold or the flu? No one knows for sure, as it is extremely hard to count exactly how many viruses exist in the nose during a cold or the flu. For medical research purposes, scientists use a special unit, known as 50 percent tissue culture infectious dose ($TCID_{50}$), to determine how many infectious particles are in nasal secretions. It is the quantity of the virus that will produce a cytopathic (cell change) effect in 50 percent of the tissue cultures inoculated.

The World Health Organization (WHO) and the U.S. Center for Disease Control and Prevention (CDC) recommend using a "nasal wash" to collect specimens for diagnosis of viral respiratory tract infections. Other methods used to collect these specimens include nasopharyngeal aspirate, nasal swab, throat swab, and nasopharyngeal swab; however, a nasal wash is considered the gold standard method because it is generally a more reliable and sensitive method to collect viruses from the nasal cavities. Here is a brief overview of how to collect a nasal-wash specimen:

Patients sit in a comfortable position with their heads tilted slightly backward. Patients are advised to keep the pharynx closed by saying "K" while a medical professional, such as a nurse, applies the washing fluid (usually normal saline) to the nostril. With a transfer pipette, 1.0 to 1.5 milliliters (mL) of washing fluid is placed in one nostril at a time. Patients then tilt their heads forward and let the washing fluid flow into a specimen cup or a Petri dish. The process is repeated with the alternate nostril until a total of 10 to 15 mL of washing fluid has been used. Depending on what type of virus is in the nasal cavities, the quantity of the virus can vary from 10 $TCID_{50}$ to 100,000 $TCID_{50}$ in 1 mL of the washing fluid.

In other words, through a simple mathematical calculation, using 10 milliliters (mL) solution could potentially remove about one million viruses from the nose. Theoretically, the severer the symptoms, the more viruses wash out through this procedure.

Medical professionals have practiced this nasal wash procedure for more than 50 years. It is a time-tested method of removing viruses and usually, if not always, the washing fluid has detectable viruses if the patients were infected.

A typical nasal wash uses about 10 mL of solution. When 240 mL of NasalCare® solution is used to perform the nasal cleanse, image how much more viruses can be removed from the body! It cannot be said that 240 mL of solution would be 24 times more effective than the 10 mL solution, but the much larger volume of solution can reach a larger area of the inner surface of the nasal cavities and can rinse the surface for a longer time and with more solution. The inner surface of the nasal cavities will be much cleaner than if only using 10 mL.

The hope is that people with asthma will decide to perform an effective nasal irrigation to remove these cold viruses from their nasal cavities. After regularly performing this effective nasal cleansing, virtually all recently inhaled or existing viruses are removed. When that happens, the viruses will not be available to trigger an asthma attack.

Know the Risks of Catching a Cold Virus

When working in a cubicle, co-workers often cough and sneeze a lot during the non-allergy season. This increases the chance of inhaling cold viruses, which can aggravate attacks in those who have asthma. Airplanes are an obvious place to inhale cold and/or flu viruses with so many people coughing and sneezing in an enclosed area. Now, people with asthma can proactively control their exposure risk by using an AsthmaCare™ Kit to get rid of any cold viruses that are inhaled on a daily basis. This way, a cold or flu can be prevented altogether.

It is easy to see how an infection spreads, especially in daycare centers, during the first two weeks of school, or during the first two weeks of training as a new solder.

Children in daycare centers give infections to each other. They drool, and their noses often drip mucus. Then, they touch each other and touch all the shared toys, spreading infection. Also, because they are constantly in contact with children who carry many different types of cold viruses, staff members are infected with these same viruses. Unfortunately, the staff members are not immune to these viruses, so they become sick themselves and pass them on to their own families.

Daycare workers can now protect themselves by performing a nasal cleansing on a regular basis. Since cold and/or flu symptoms generally appear one to three days after exposure to the virus, there is a window of opportunity to perform an effective nasal cleansing before the infection can even start.

The cold and/or flu virus can spread easily and strike an entire community all at once. Performing a nasal cleansing every day can help to prevent the spread of these viruses. Thus, there will be less of a chance to trigger an asthma attack.

It is also commonly known that pregnant women are more susceptible to catching a cold, which can trigger an asthma flare-up. Cold viruses have also been linked to abnormalities in the fetus. Because of safety concerns for the fetus, pregnant women are particularly advised not to take many medications. Using an AsthmaCare™ Kit can effectively remove cold viruses from the body without harming the fetus. The homeopathic oral spray is safe for both a pregnant woman and the fetus.

How to Start Nasal Cleansing Sooner

It is well documented that asthma flare-ups are more frequent during the cold season. The best practice is to keep one AsthmaCare™ Kit at home and one in the office. That way, anyone can perform a nasal cleanse as soon as possible after exposure to someone who is coughing and sneezing.

Where to Get an AsthmaCare™ Kit

The AsthmaCare™ Kit is sold over-the-counter at many stores. The AsthmaCare™ Kit is also available from the manufacturer by calling toll free at 1-888-658-8108, or visiting the manufacturer's online store at www.nasalcleanse.com.

How to Use AsthmaCare™ Kit

Here are the easy-to-follow directions for using the AsthmaCare™ Kit:

A. Basic Nasal Cleansing Procedures:

1) Wash hands. Remove the clear dust cover, and then remove the cap from the bottle. Open one NasalCare® Nasal Rinse Mix packet and pour all the contents into the bottle.

2) Fill the bottle with sterilized warm water (about body temperature) to the 8-ounce (240 mL) line. Make sure the gasket is securely within the cap and the tube is tightly inserted into the small connector in the cap. Screw the cap onto the bottle tightly. Shake the bottle several times to dissolve the mixture. To keep the solution from spilling out, use the tip of a finger to block the opening of the nostril fitting.

3) Bend forward over a sink, as if brushing the teeth. Place the nostril fitting snugly into one nostril. Breathe through the mouth, not the nose, to perform nasal irrigation. Squeeze and release the bottle gently to allow the solution to flow into the nostril on one side, and let the washing solution flow out from the other nostril. Squeeze and release repeatedly about every half second.

4. How to Avoid or Remove Asthma Triggers

Doing so makes the cleansing process more efficient and relaxing. Do not squeeze the bottle all the way in one motion or squeeze for too long. Otherwise, the hand pump will not function properly.

4) Gently blow nose to remove the mucus.

5) Repeat steps 3 and 4 in the other nostril.

B. Alternative Cleansing Procedures

1) During Step 3, if the left and right nostrils are not connected, let the solution run into the nostril and then flow out from the mouth; making sure to inhale through the nose, then spit the solution into the sink.

2) Even if the left and right nostrils are connected through the nasopharynx, the liquid can be allowed to run from the nostril into mouth. This way, both the nasopharynx and oropharynx are cleansed.

3) Initially, some patients may be nervous about having water enter their nasal cavity, perhaps recalling unpleasant memories of water entering their noses while swimming. However, since the AsthmaCare™ solution has been carefully designed to suit the sensitive lining of the nose, nasal cleanse with the AsthmaCare™ Kit is comfortable, even pleasant, as reported by some patients.

A Most Complete Nasal Cleansing Procedure

To have a complete nasal cavity, nasopharynx and oropharynx cleansing, try the following procedure after mastering the basic procedure.

1) Gently pump the solution into one nostril, letting about ¼ of the solution (about 2 ounces) in the bottle to flow out from the other nostril; then gently blow nose. This is to cleanse the left nasal passage, sinuses, nasopharynx, and finally, the right side of the nasal passage.

2) Gently pump 2 more ounces of solution into the other nostril, letting it flow out from the opposite nostril, and then gently

blow the nose. This is to cleanse the right nasal passage, sinuses, nasopharynx from the other direction, and finally, the left side of the nasal passage.

3) Gently pump another 2 ounces of solution into the left side of the nostril. When that side of the nasal cavity feels full, inhale the liquid through the nose so the solution enters the mouth. Spit the solution out into the sink. This will cleanse the left nasal passage, left sinuses, nasopharynx, and then the left side of the oropharynx and throat.

4) Gently pump the last 2 ounces of solution into the right nostril; when that side of the nasal cavity feels full, inhale the liquid through the nose so the solution enters the mouth. Spit the solution out into the sink. This will cleanse the right nasal passage, right sinuses, nasopharynx, and then the right side of the oropharynx and throat.

Removing Residual Liquid

It is common to have a small amount of liquid left in the nasal cavity, mainly in the maxillary sinuses, since the floor of this pair of sinuses is lower than the floor of the nasal cavity.

To drain the residual liquid from the sinuses, bend over, point the nose towards the knees, and then gently shake the head left to right a few times. Raise head slowly as some of the residual liquid drips out. Repeat this action several more times to remove all the residual liquid.

Maintenance after Each Use

After each nasal cleansing, fill the bottle with tap water and replace the cap. Pump water through it a few times, so that the entire liquid passage is completely rinsed. Rinse the outside of the irrigator, especially the part that fits into the nostril, since that is the only piece to have touched the nose. Let all the rinsed parts air dry for the next use.

Initially, nasal irrigation may seem a little difficult to do, as it requires a few steps to assemble before each use. However, after just one use, it is actually very simple and easy to do. Many users have shared that using the AsthmaCare™ Kit is easier than using neti pots.

How to Use the AsthmaCare™ Oral Spray

The AsthmaCare™ Oral Spray is formulated with 23 active homeopathic ingredients, designed to reduce the severity of asthma symptoms and decrease airway sensitivity that is more susceptible to asthma triggers.

For best results, use regularly every day, particularly at the onset of non-severe symptoms. If severe asthma symptoms are present, consult a physician immediately and use a rescue inhaler. Below is how to use the oral spray:

1) Spray 1 dose each time. Use 3 sprays for adults and 2 sprays for children in the mouth, on the inside of the cheeks, on the roof of the mouth and on the gums.

2) Retain for 15 seconds before swallowing.

3) Repeat every 2 to 4 hours; spraying up to 6 doses per day as needed, until symptoms subside.

4) After using this homeopathic spray, do not eat or drink anything for 15 minutes to allow the oral cavity membrane to absorb the spray.

5) Other medications can be taken if needed, as this homeopathic spray has no known interactions with any other medications.

Professional medical care should always be sought for any asthma flare-up. Please consult a physician before trying any other methods to control asthma flare-ups.

5. Drugs to Treat Asthma

Asthma medication plays a key role in gaining good control over asthma. Asthma is a chronic disease that involves inflammation of the airways superimposed with recurrent episodes of decreased airflow, mucus production, and cough. Choosing the proper asthma medication is crucial in avoiding asthma attacks and living an active life.

The contents of this chapter as well as other chapters are for informational purposes only and are not meant as specific medical advice. Please contact a physician to discuss specific asthma treatment needs.

People with asthma should discuss effective long-term asthma care plans with their physicians. Below are these common statements. If the answer is "YES" to any of the statements below, share them with a physician.

In the last 3 months, I:

1) Had an asthma flare-up and needed to see a doctor

2) Need to use a rescue inhaler more than twice a week

3) Have had asthma symptoms, like wheezing or shortness of breath more often

4) Had sudden asthma symptoms and had to get emergency treatment by a doctor

5) Had to take an oral steroid medicine for asthma

6) Had woken up at night more often to use a rescue inhaler

Treatment plans using asthma medication generally focuses on controlling inflammation and preventing chronic symptoms, such as coughing or breathlessness at night or early morning; taking asthma medication as prescribed to treat asthma attacks when they occur; avoiding asthma triggers by monitoring daily asthma symptoms in an asthma diary; and monitoring peak flows with daily asthma tests.

Different Types of Asthma Medication

There are two general types of asthma medication that provide either long-term control or quick relief of symptoms.

Anti-inflammatory drugs are the first type; these are the most important type of therapy for most people with asthma because these medications prevent asthma attacks on an ongoing basis. Steroids, also called "corticosteroids," are vital anti-inflammatory medications for people suffering from asthma because they reduce swelling and mucus production in the airways. As a result, airways are less sensitive and less likely to react to triggers.

Bronchodilators are the second type. These drugs relieve the symptoms of asthma by relaxing the muscle bands that tighten around the airways during an attack. This action rapidly opens the airways, letting more air in and out of the lungs. As a result, breathing is improved and more oxygen enters the blood. Bronchodilators also help clear mucus from the lungs. As the airways open, the mucus moves more freely and coughed out more easily.

These asthma medications can be administered in different ways. Successful treatment generally results in an active and normal life. If asthma symptoms are not under control, contact a physician for advice about different asthma medication options

Long-term control asthma medications are taken daily over an extended period to achieve and maintain control of persistent asthma. Persistent asthma is a special type of asthma that causes symptoms more than twice a week and recurrent attacks that interfere with daily living and working activities.

Long-Term Control Asthma Medications

Some of the asthma medications that are available for long-term control of symptoms include :

1) **Corticosteroids.** The inhaled form of corticosteroids is the anti-inflammatory drug of choice for persistent asthma.

2) **Long acting beta-agonists.** These bronchodilators are often used in conjunction with an anti-inflammatory drug.

3) **Theophylline.** This bronchodilator is used along with an anti-inflammatory drug to prevent nighttime symptoms.

4) **Leukotriene modifiers.** These are an alternative to steroids and mast cell stabilizers.

5) **Omalizumab.** This injectable medication can be used when inhaled steroids for asthma fail to control symptoms in people with moderate to severe asthma who also have allergies.

Quick-Relief Asthma Medications

These asthma medications are used to provide prompt relief of asthma attack symptoms, such as cough, chest tightness, and wheezing. These include:

1) **Short acting beta-agonists.** These bronchodilators are the drug of choice to relieve asthma attacks and prevent exercise-induced asthma symptoms.

2) **Anti-cholinergics.** This is another bronchodilator that can be used in conjunction with short-acting beta-agonists, or as an alternative medication.

3) **Systemic corticosteroids.** These anti-inflammatory drugs are used in an emergency to gain rapid control of an attack while initiating other treatments and to help speed recovery.

Asthma medications come in many forms, such as inhalers, nebulizers, injectables, and pills. Since some asthma m-edications can be taken together, some inhalers contain a combination of two different medications. These devices allow delivery of both medications simultaneously from one device, shortening treatment times and decreasing the number of inhalers needed to treat asthma symptoms.

Over-the-Counter Asthma Drugs

Primatene Mist® and Bronkaid® are very common over-the-counter (OTC) asthma drugs. They both work like a bronchodilator, relaxing the muscles around the airways. They provide short-term relief (20-30 minutes), but do not control asthma symptoms long-term or prevent asthma attacks. People with high blood pressure, diabetes, thyroid disease, or heart disease should not take Primatene Mist® or Bronkaid®. Unfortunately, many people misuse or overuse these asthma treatments. These OTC drugs are not meant for long-term use, yet some people use them every day to relieve asthma symptoms. Because they do not control asthma, people who take them may not be receiving proper treatment for their asthma.

If a person with asthma is using an OTC asthma drugs and still experiencing frequent asthma symptoms, they should talk to their physicians about other ways to control their asthma. Physicians should also know if their patients with asthma who are already taking prescribed asthma drugs, are also using OTC medications to prevent overmedication.

Asthma cannot be cured and symptoms can be hard to control. Additionally, how often to take asthma medication depends on the severity of the attacks and the frequency of the symptoms. For example, if asthma symptoms take place only during a certain time of year, like allergy season, then medications to control the symptoms are only necessary during that period. However, this is somewhat unusual, and most people with asthma need to take medications every day.

Manage Your Asthma with Medications

Asthma medications are the foundation of good asthma control. People with asthma should become knowledgeable about the medications they are taking. It is also important to know what medications are included in their asthma action plan, when these medications should be taken, their expected results, and what to do when they fail to relieve asthma symptoms.

Below are some general guidelines to help people with asthma to adhere to their asthma action plans:

1) Never run out of asthma medications. Call the pharmacy or physician's office at least 48 hours before running out of

any asthma medications. It is good to keep pharmacy phone numbers, prescription numbers, and medication names and doses readily available to call in refills easily.

2) Refer to the asthma action plan prescribed by a physician when deciding how or when to use asthma drugs. Physicians design the plan to achieve the best asthma control possible; patients must understand and follow the plan exactly.

3) Wash hands prior to preparing or taking asthma medications.

4) Take the necessary time to prepare medications properly. Double-check the name and dosage of all asthma medications before using them.

5) Keep all asthma medications stored according to the instructions given with the prescription.

6) Check liquid medications often. If they have changed color or formed crystals, throw them away and get new ones.

7) Inform physicians about any other medications, either prescription or OTC, that are taken. Some medications can affect the actions of asthma medications when taken together.

8) Most asthma medications are safe. However, side effects can occur and vary depending on the medication and dose. Ask a physician or pharmacist about the side effects. Report any unusual or severe side effects to a physician immediately.

6. Alternative Approaches to Treat Asthma

To help relieve their asthma, many people try complementary and alternative asthma such as herbal or homeopathic remedies, breathing exercises, and yoga. Researchers are investigating whether these types of treatments really work on asthma and are safe for use during an attack. Below are commonly used complementary and alternative treatments for asthma.

Acupuncture

Acupuncture involves the insertion of very thin needles into the skin at specific points on the body. Acupuncture originated in China thousands of years ago, and its popularity has grown significantly in other parts of the world. Some studies suggest that asthma symptoms may improve with acupuncture, but there is still not enough clear evidence to be certain. If a person with asthma decides to try acupuncture, they should only work with an experienced, licensed acupuncturist or a medical doctor who practices acupuncture. When delivered by trained practitioners, acupuncture is relatively low risk.

Breathing exercises

Breathing techniques for asthma have been around for years, but many health providers remain skeptical about their effectiveness, as they do not seem to improve the underlying allergic reaction that causes asthma symptoms. Nonetheless, in a number of studies, people who did breathing exercises reported improved symptoms. Breathing methods vary, but generally they involve learning how to:

1) Take breaths less often

2) Take slower breaths

3) Breathe through the nose rather than the mouth

4) Use the abdominal muscles to take deep "belly breaths", also known as diaphragmatic breathing

A few breathing techniques used for asthma include the Buteyko breathing technique and yoga breathing (pranayama). Some methods also offer advice about stress reduction, medication use, nutrition and general health. Some clinics and researchers offer breathing technique instruction as part of asthma treatment, either face-to-face or via video or Internet.

Herbal remedies

Herbal remedies have been used for thousands of years to treat lung disorders and are still considered a primary asthma treatment in many countries. Some have shown promise in research, but more studies are still needed to find out for certain what works and what is safe. Herbs that have shown at least some promise in treating asthma symptoms include:

- Butterbur
- Dried ivy
- Ginkgo extract
- Tylophora indica
- French maritime pine bark extract (pycnogenol)
- Indian frankincense (Boswellia serrata)
- Choline

Blends of different types of herbs are commonly used in traditional Chinese, Indian and Japanese medicine. Certain combinations of herbs may be more effective than taking one herbal remedy by itself.

Use caution when taking herbal remedies and always discuss the use of any new herb or dietary supplement with a physician. Consider these concerns before taking any herbal remedy:

- **Quality and dose.** Until recently, the quality of herbal and dietary supplements sold in the United States was often suspect. Things have improved with the introduction of guidelines from the Food and Drug Administration (FDA). The guidelines help ensure that manufacturers accurately indicate on the label what is in the bottle. While this is a significant step forward, it is still recommended to research different brands.

- **Side effects.** Side effects caused by herbal supplements can range from minor to severe, and depend on the herb and the dose taken. Be especially cautious of herbal asthma remedies that contain ephedra-like substances, which may cause high

6. Alternative Approaches to Treat Asthma

blood pressure and are linked to heart attack and stroke. Examples include ma-huang (banned in the United States) and bitter orange.

- **Drug interactions.** Certain herbal remedies can interact with other medications. Always consult a physician before taking an herbal remedy.

These concerns do not necessarily mean trying an herbal treatment is a bad idea; care just needs to be taken when considering adding herbal remedies to an existing asthma treatment plan. Speak with a physician before taking an herbal remedy to make sure it is safe for use.

Inspiration muscle training

This technique helps strengthen lung muscles with a series of breathing exercises. It is sometimes used for other lung diseases, such as chronic obstructive pulmonary disease (COPD), and after certain types of surgery. These exercises definitely strengthen the muscles of the lungs, but there is not enough proof to say whether they help with asthma, specifically.

Massage and chiropractic treatment

Although some claim that these treatments help, there is no evidence that physical manipulation of the spine or muscles reduces asthma symptoms.

Relaxation therapy

Relaxation therapy techniques include meditation, biofeedback, hypnosis and progressive muscle relaxation. It is unclear whether any of these techniques directly help with asthma, but they do seem to reduce stress and promote a sense of well-being.

Vitamins and supplements

More research is needed to determine whether vitamins or other nutrients may help ease asthma symptoms in people who have a deficiency. Three that seem promising include:

1) **Antioxidants.** People with severe asthma appear to have decreased levels of these protective nutrients naturally found in fruits and vegetables. Antioxidants such as vitamin C, vitamin A, and magnesium may have some effect on asthma by boosting the immune system.

2) **Omega-3 fatty acids.** Found in several types of fish, healthy oils containing omega-3s may reduce the inflammation that leads to asthma symptoms, but the verdict is still out. They also appear to have a number of other health benefits. It is not yet clear whether omega-3s from vegetable sources have the same beneficial effects as the omega-3s found in fish.

3) **Vitamin D.** Vitamin D deficiency is associated with increased airway hyper-responsiveness, decreased lung functions, and inferior asthma control. Vitamin D deficiency is more common with obesity and in African American ethnicity.

Use of antioxidants, omega-3 fatty acids or vitamin D can complement a prescribed asthma treatment plan as they may have some anti-inflammatory properties. However, they should never be used as an alternative to prescribed medication. Asthma is a serious and sometimes life-threatening disease that requires medical treatment. Always discuss use of supplements with an allergist or physician.

A multivitamin or supplement pill may help add nutrients to a diet, but the best way to ensure adequate nutrition is to eat a varied diet rich in fresh, unprocessed foods.

46 You Too Can be Free from Asthma

7. Asthma Prevention

Asthma symptoms can be substantially reduced by avoiding known allergens and irritants. If someone with asthma is sensitive to dust mites, encasing mattresses and pillows in allergen-impermeable covers, removing carpets from bedrooms and by vacuuming regularly can reduce the frequency of attacks. Exposure to dust mites and moles can be reduced by lowering indoor humidity. If a person is allergic to an animal that cannot be removed from the home, the animal should be kept out of the person's bedroom. Filtering material can be placed over the heating outlets to trap animal dander. Exposure to cigarette smoke, air pollution, industrial dusts, and irritating fumes should also be avoided.

With all of the possible asthma triggers that are in the environment, can someone remain asthma-free for a long period? Yes, it is! Some medical and non-medical approaches have been very successful. For example, if people with asthma get a flu shot, their asthma attacks that winter are reduced significantly. The same applies to those who regularly get allergy shots. If people with asthma are treated with antibodies against certain inflammation factors, their asthma flare-ups decrease. Boosting the immune system can help reduce asthma attacks by suppressing viral infections. Using homeopathic products can also help diminish the frequency and severity of asthma. Finally, a simple nasal cavity cleanse can also physically eliminate these viral and allergic triggers; resulting in less recurrent attacks. There are so many ways to protect against asthma attacks and enjoy freedom from asthma. So how and why are these approaches so beneficial to people with asthma?

Flu Vaccination

As the influenza virus infection can trigger an asthma attack, getting the flu may not only make asthma flare-up, it may also cause a severe enough attack to require a visit to the ER and subsequent hospitalization. Getting a flu shot helps to prevent all of these complications. According to the CDC, anyone with asthma over the age of 6 months should get a flu shot every year. Despite this recommendation, many people do not get flu shots. Adults with asthma are at a higher risk of developing complications after contracting the influenza virus, yet only one-third of all asthmatic adults receive the flu vaccine annually (CDC 2011). Although a small percentage of people could have some side effects from a flu shot, people with asthma should have an annual flu vaccination to help prevent the flu from triggering an asthma attack. The ratio of benefit to risk is overwhelming for people with asthma.

Allergy Shots

As is well documented, allergies trigger most cases of asthma. As a result, if allergies are under control, then fewer asthma attacks will occur. Immunotherapy, or allergy shots, is very effective at controlling allergy symptoms. These shots are injections of a small quantity of the specific allergens that trigger asthma attacks in a person. Overtime, and after subsequent injections, the person with asthma develops a tolerance to these triggers, resulting in improved allergy symptoms and a lesser risk of asthma attacks. Consult a physician to discuss whether allergies could be the cause of asthma attacks.

Using Antibodies to Reduce Eosinophilic Asthma Attack

A significant portion of the asthmatic patients with severe asthma have what is called eosinophilic asthma, in which inflammatory cells, called eosinophils, cause swelling of lung airways. Standard asthma treatment with inhaled steroids is not effective, so these patients take oral steroids, which have many side effects. Recently, a group of medical researchers reported that an experimental drug, known as mepolizumab, when given intravenously, reduced asthma outbreaks by almost 50 percent in people with a special type of hard-to-treat asthma. How did the drug do this? The new antibody blocked the production of eosinophils and reduced the frequency of severe asthma outbreaks, which may decrease the need for steroids. For sure, this is a promising new drug therapy. However, it will take a few more years for the experimental drug to be approved for use for this special type of asthma. In addition, although this new antibody effectively reduced asthma attacks, it did not improve symptoms or lung function, so it is not a cure. This drug needs to be injected repeatedly for a long time and the cost is still unknown.

New Anti-IgE Drug to Reduce Asthma Attacks

Immunoglobulin E (IgE) plays a key role in triggering asthma attacks. Respiratory viruses and allergies work together or individually to raise the IgE level in the airway to prompt an attack. Using an antibody against IgE can help to eliminate this key component, and possibly prevent seasonal asthma attacks very effectively. A new clinical study used a new antibody to knock out IgE that resulted in a significant reduction in asthma attacks. A national research team of clinical researchers led by Dr. William Busse, reported that treatment with the anti-IgE antibody decreased the milder year-round asthma symptoms among the young people, who had allergies and lived in the inner cities of the United States, which is considered a very high-risk group of patients. The goal of their clinical trial was to see if adding the special antibody against IgE would reduce the number of severe attacks and the number of days participants had asthma symptoms (UWHealth website).

This treatment shuts down IgE, the protein that triggers allergic reactions. In the study, half of the participants received anti-IgE antibody, and the other half a placebo, injected under the skin every two to four weeks over 60 weeks, along with standard asthma treatment. At the end of the study, the analysis showed no seasonal spikes in asthma attacks among participants who received anti-IgE antibody. That group also had a 25 percent reduction in asthma-symptom days, a 30 percent reduction in asthma attacks and a nearly 15 percent reduction in use of inhaled corticosteroids when compared with those who received placebo. The anti-IgE drug group also had a 75 percent reduction in hospital admissions of the asthmatic patients. Their results are very encouraging and serve to help physicians and patients to plan for asthma management when the drug is approved in the future. Again, it will take several years to receive approval for this new drug.

Anti-Interleukin 13 (IL-13) Antibody

Another experimental new drug, Tralokinumab, is a human monoclonal antibody that targets the cytokine interleukin 13, and is designed for the treatment of asthma and inflammatory diseases (Kopf 2010). It was reported that this drug candidate has a good efficacy signal and has progressed to Phase Two clinical trial. Again, it will take many years to receive approval for this new drug.

A Combinational Therapy

Until these experimental drugs are approved, there is an OTC product to prevent asthma. The 2-in-1 combinational therapy offered under the DrHealing™ name brand, called the AsthmaCare™ Kit, is now available. The AsthmaCare™ Kit can be used to cleanse away these asthma triggers and reduce the severity of attacks. The Kit will be described in more detail in Chapter 9.

7. Asthma Prevention

8. Homeopathy for Treating Asthma

When "asthma homeopathy" was typed into a Google search on October 14, 2012, 3,030,000 results were listed. This is very impressive even with so much information now available online. This also shows that homeopathy is becoming quite popular.

According to the FDA's guidelines, homeopathic drugs are over-the-counter (OTC) medicines, which mean they can be purchased at a pharmacy without a physician's prescription. Homeopathy aims to stimulate the body's self-healing response by using a tiny harmful substance to prime the body so it can challenge infections and inflammation more effectively.

The very small doses of homeopathic substances that are used are very beneficial; taking homeopathic substances in large amounts could cause severe harm. The key is using a "tiny amount". The poison or toxic substance is diluted to an extremely low concentration, such as one part per billion ($1/10^9$). At that low amount, the substance has lost its poisonous or toxic effect. The body, however, senses its presence, and then develops a defense system to protect the body from any harm if the poison or toxin were to be introduced into the body at a larger amount. In the case of asthma, homeopathic remedies are made from substances that would cause asthma symptoms at a larger amount. Since so many substances can cause asthma symptoms, the more ingredients used in the homeopathic remedies, the broader protection it will provide.

Homeopaths have a long history of successful allergy treatment, and they have made some important contributions to the present understanding of allergies. In fact, it was a British homeopath in 1871, named C.H. Blackely, who first noted that seasonal sneezing and nasal discharge were the result of exposure to pollen. An American homeopath, Dr. Grant L. Selfridge, was one of three physicians to start the organization that later became the current American Academy of Allergy.

There are concerns that homeopathic remedies lack scientific evidence to support their efficacy. The doses of the homeopathic ingredients used are so small that homeopaths and modern scientists acknowledge that there should be no remaining molecules of the original substance after dilution. Homeopaths theorize that the unique pharmacological process of serial dilution with vigorous shaking in between each dilution may create an even more potent medicine. New concepts in physics, especially relating to chaos theory and fractals, suggest that homeopathic medicine is best understood through these innovative concepts of science.

Although homeopathic medicine is little known in the U.S., it is very popular throughout the world, especially Europe. Approximately 40% of French physicians and 20% of German physicians prescribe homeopathic medicines. Over 40% of British physicians refer patients of homeopaths, and almost 50% of Dutch physicians consider these natural medicines to be effective.

Based on what experts in homeopathy experienced, homeopathic therapy can achieve the followings:

1) Reduce significantly the frequency of asthmatic attacks

2) Reduce significantly the severity of asthmatic attacks

3) Reduce the duration of asthma attacks

4) Reduce the need for bronchodilators, cortisone and antibiotics (in case of infections), in many patients

5) In children, homeopathic treatment may eliminate the need for other medications.

Those who do not use homeopathy for asthma are deprived of the wonderful benefits of it. Homeopathic experts recommend homeopathy during all stages of asthma. Please go to https://www.pramilahomeopathy.com for more information.

As stated on this website, this group of homeopathic doctors has treated people with asthma successfully for more than 35 years. Their individualized treatment has helped more than 10,000 patients overcome their disabilities due to asthma and lead normal lives.

Following the principle of "evidence-based medicine," homeopathy is the one type of medicine that tries to cure the disease, instead of

8. Homeopathy for Treating Asthma

trying to provide just symptomatic relief. While dealing with a case of asthma, a homeopath not only observes the symptoms of the disease but also studies the medical history, family history, and the physical and psychological characteristics of a person. This helps to find other possible causes, precipitating factors, hereditary tendencies, etc., that may contribute to a person's asthma attacks. Of special interest to a homeopath is the history of suppression of skin disease. Homeopaths believe that when there is a tendency or predisposition for a disease, it first manifests on the less vital organs, towards the outside of the body, like the skin. If the manifestation is suppressed, the disease then shifts inwards, towards the more vital organs, like lungs, heart, brain etc.

Both homeopaths and allopaths (conventional medical doctors) recognize that in children, asthma is often preceded by eczema. This fact is written in all textbooks of modern medicine. They say that children often "move-out" of eczema, an inflammation of the skin characterized by reddening, itching and the formation of scaly or crusty patches that may leak fluid, and "move-into" asthma. However, they are unable to make a direct correlation. Homeopaths believe that the suppression of eczema with topical preparations does not cure the disease or sensitivity of the person, but merely drives the disease inwards.

Now, after ascertaining the symptoms and the cause, the homeopath tries to find a medicine that matches the symptoms as well as the general characteristics of the person. The right medicine is then selected, developed, and administered to the patient.

It is often observed by homeopaths that when the right medicine is given, the asthma disappears, but the old eczema often reappears for some time, before finally disappearing itself. This reappearance of old symptoms is viewed as a reversal of the disease process and is considered a very good prognostic sign by homeopaths.

Homoeopathic medicines may offer a permanent cure in asthma by decreasing the hyperactivity of immune cells and restraining the individual's immune response against allergens, thus decreasing their hypersensitivity towards triggering stimuli. The development of allergic conditions is multi-factorial and depends upon interaction between susceptible receptors on the immune cell surface and these environmental factors. Homeopathy, like immunotherapy, can alter this hypersensitivity. Thus, homoeopathy with the right ingredients offers excellent results.

There are many medicines in homeopathy for treating asthma and it is not possible to list them all. The selection of medicine varies from patient to patient. For treating a group of patients with asthma with an OTC homeopathic drug, many more kinds of homeopathic ingredients should be used to cover as many causes as possible.

The AsthmaCare™ Kit is a 2-in-1 therapy that includes a homeopathic oral spray with a nasal cleansing system. The spray is formulated with 23 active homeopathic ingredients. When compared with other homeopathic remedies, this homeopathic medicine has the most number of active ingredients. Each of these 23 ingredients has its unique therapeutic effects:

1) **Antimonium Tartaricum**: Its therapeutic application has been confined largely to the treatment of respiratory diseases, rattling of mucus with little expectoration has been a guiding symptom.

2) **Aralia Racemosa**: This remedy is for asthmatic conditions, with cough aggravated on lying down. Drenching sweat during sleep. Extreme sensitiveness to draughts. Dry cough coming on after first sleep, about middle of night. Asthma on lying down at night with spasmodic cough; worse after first sleep, with tickling in throat. Constriction of chest; feels as if a foreign body were in throat. Obstruction is worse in spring. Hay fever; frequent sneezing. Rawness and burning behind sternum.

3) **Arsenicum Album**: For treating aggravated breathlessness, exhaustion, with nightly aggravation. A person needing this homeopathic asthma remedy may often feel a combination of exhaustion and uneasiness. Breathing problems are exacerbated when supine, better when upright. The person often finds that ease of breathing deteriorates at night, accompanied by wheezing and a constant thirst. He/she may also experience violent chills accompanied by shivering; heat may bring relief.

4) **Blatta Orientalis**: A remedy for asthma. Especially when associated with bronchitis. Cough with dyspnoea in bronchitis and phthisis. Acts best in stout and corpulent patients.

5) **Bryonia Alba**: Acts on all serous membranes and the viscera they contain. Aching in every muscle. The pain here is a stitching, tearing; worse by motion, especially in the chest; worse pressure. Mucous membranes are all dry.

6) **Carbo Vegetabilis**: This homeopathic asthma treatment is generally prescribed when the person has violent bouts of coughing, which may cause a gag reflex to set in. Extremities might be cold, but there is a need for air or breeze. Feels dyspeptic, burping gives relief.

7) **Chamomilla**: This is most often prescribed for asthma attacks that are brought on by emotional stress, anxiety or over excitement. The person displays behavior that is irritable, angry and hypersensitive. In some cases, this is accompanied by a racking cough.

8) **Drosera Rotundifolia**: Affects markedly the respiratory organs. Considered by Dr. Hahnemann to be a principal remedy for whooping cough. Spasmodic, irritated cough, the paroxysms following each other very rapidly; can scarcely breathe; chokes. Cough very deep and hoarse, and becomes worse after midnight; yellow expectoration, with bleeding from nose and mouth; retching. Deep, hoarse voice; hoarseness; laryngitis. Rough, scraping sensation deep in the fauces and soft palate. Sensation as if crumbs were in the throat, of feather in larynx. Laryngeal phthisis, with rapid emaciation. Harassing and titilating cough in children-not at all through the day, but commences as soon as the head touches the pillow at night. Clergyman's sore throat, with rough, scraping, dry sensation deep in the fauces; voice hoarse, deep, toneless, cracked, requires exertion to speak. Asthma when talking, with contraction of the throat at every word uttered.

9) **Eupatorium Perfoliatum**: it relieves pain in limbs and muscles that accompanies some forms of febrile disease, like malaria and influenza.

10) **Histaminum Hydrochloricum**: It is primarily used to treat various allergies, including those caused by food, insect bites and pollen, and allergy symptoms such as skin irritations, nasal congestion and breathing difficulties.

11) **Ipecacuanha**: Its chief action is on the ramifications of the pneumogastric nerve, producing spasmodic irritation in chest and stomach. Morphia habit. The principal feature of Ipecacuanha is to suppress persistent nausea and vomiting.
12) **Kali Carbonicum**: For treating thick, fluent, yellow discharge. Post-nasal dripping. Sore, scurfy nostrils; bloody nasal mucus. Crusty nasal openings. Nosebleed on washing face in morning. Ulcerated nostrils.

13) **Lobelia Inflata**: It is a vasomotor stimulant; increases the activity of all vegetative processes; spends its force mainly upon the pneumogastric nerve, producing a depressed relaxed condition with oppression of the chest and epigastrium, impeded respiration, nausea and vomiting.

14) **Natrum Sulphuricum**: For treating nasal disorders, nasal catarrh, with thick, yellow discharge and salty mucus. When asthma attacks are precipitated by mould and dampness, this homeopathy remedy is especially efficacious.

15) **Nux vomica**: For treating nasal disorders, such as stuffed up, at night especially. Stuffy colds, snuffles, after exposure to dry, cold atmosphere; worse, in warm room. Persons feeling constricted in the chest and stomach, brought on by having spicy food, alcohol and sweets. Warmth and sleep along with this remedy bring relief.

16) **Phosporus**: For treating irritants, inflames and degenerates mucous membranes, irritates and inflames serous membranes.

17) **Pothos Foetidus**: For asthmatic complaints; worse from inhaling any dust. Erratic spasmodic pains. Millar's asthma.

18) **Pulsatilla Nigricans**: For treating great sensitiveness, mucous membranes disorder, discharges thick, bland, and yellowish-green. Excessive warmth especially indoors along with and heavily spiced food bring on wheezing because of exertion and chest congestion. This remedy is useful for children suffering from asthma.

19) **Quebracho**: For stimulating respiratory centers, increasing oxidation and excretion of carbonic acid. Pulmonary stenosis. Thrombosis of pulmonary artery.

20) **Sambucus Nigra**: Acts especially on the respiratory organs. Dry coryza of infants, snuffles, oedematous swellings. Profuse sweat accompanies many affections. Relieving sore throat and fever.

21) **Spongia Tosta**: A remedy especially marked in the symptoms of the respiratory organs, cough, croup, etc.

22) **Sticta Pulmonaria**: For treating a set of symptoms like coryza, bronchial catarrh and influenza, together with nervous and rheumatic disturbances. There is a general feeling of dullness and malaise, as when a cold is coming on, dull, heavy pressure in forehead, catarrhal conjunctivitis, etc. Rheumatic stiffness of neck.

23) **Urtica Urens**: A remedy for agalactia and lithiasis. Profuse discharge from mucous surfaces. Enuresis and urticaria. Spleen affections. Antidotes ill effects of eating shellfish. Symptoms return at the same time every year. Gout and uric acid diathesis. Favors elimination.

The efficacy of homeopathic remedies differs according to the exact condition of a person's health status. Generally, asthma improvement begins within the first week and lasts about four weeks.

Be advised that in case of a severe asthma condition or attack evidenced by extreme breathlessness, paleness, cyanotic lips, and the possibility of losing consciousness, seek help from a conventional physician immediately.

9. Treat and Prevent Asthma Using 2-in-1 Therapy

The Environmental Load is Heavy

An effective approach to asthma treatment is to reduce the total environmental load that people with asthma experience. These include infectious aerosols and droplets in working or living environments, and allergens and inflammatory agents in the air, food and drink. Reducing this complicated airborne environmental load is so important for gaining asthma-free days. Can people with asthma do it? Yes, by using the AsthmaCare™ Kit to help eliminate the heavy environmental load.

The Unmet Need is Great

As evidenced from the previous chapters, asthma is a very complicated disease since so many harmful substances can trigger its attack. Particularly, many viruses, allergens and other known or unknown factors are capable of causing an asthma attack, either by acting alone or in conjunction with each other. There is no cure for asthma and it is extremely difficult to prevent or treat with existing medications because there are so many different kinds of triggers. Therefore, there is a great, unmet need for relief from asthma attacks.

The 2-in-1 Therapy

The good news is that a combinational therapy with an OTC medical device and an OTC drug brings great hope for people with asthma. The 2-in-1 combinational therapy offered under the DrHealing™ name brand, called the AsthmaCare™ Kit, is now available.

What are the unique benefits of using the AsthmaCare™ Kit? People with asthma will have the ability to:

1) Cleanse out common respiratory viruses from the upper airway. Reduced viruses in the upper airway will diminish the chance for asthma flare-ups.

2) Cleanse out common respiratory allergens, such as pollen, from the upper airway. Reduced allergens in the upper airway will also diminish the chance for asthma flare-ups.

3) Cleanse out both common respiratory viruses and allergens from the upper airway simultaneously. When both major asthma triggers are removed from the upper airway, they cannot act together to cause harm, which should reduce the chance for asthma flare-ups.

4) Cleanse out common inflammatory mediators from the upper airway. This reduced concentration of inflammatory mediators in the upper airway will decrease the sensitivity of the airway to help avoid new asthma flare-ups.

5) Prime the body with homeopathic spray to reduce the sensitivity of the airway and decrease the risk of new asthma flare-ups.

Using this 2-in-1 combinational therapy has multiple benefits because it cleanses out common viruses, allergens, and inflammatory mediators from the upper airway. These harmful substances will then have less chance to flow down to the lower airway; allowing the lower airway a chance to have a peaceful environment to begin self-healing.

It is hard to guarantee a freedom from asthma for a long time since so many asthma triggers are in the environment. These harmful substances in the environment can cause trouble anytime after inhaling them. However, by keeping the AsthmaCare™ Kit on hand all the time and cleansing the upper airway regularly, there is a better chance of reducing asthma flare-ups and diminishing the severity of asthma attacks.

Is it practical? Absolutely! Bring the AsthmaCare™ Kit to work or school to continue the combination therapy any time, as needed. It only takes about 2 minutes to complete the nasal cleanse and oral spray procedure, not much different from brushing the teeth after lunch at work.

Cleansing the nasal cavity is beneficial for other people because there will be less cold and/or flu viruses to spread. After performing a complete nasal cleanse, the mucus carrying the viruses is gone and the nasal cavities are clean, with not as many virus particles to spread around.

Since performing the nasal cleanse with the award winning nasal irrigator and using a homeopathic spray with 23 homeopathic ingredients have no side effects, the 2-in-1 combinational therapy can be used any day, at any time. It is simple and safe enough to use repeatedly.

10. Frequently Asked Questions about Asthma

Q: What is asthma?

A: The Global Initiative for Asthma, as part of the Global Strategy for Asthma Management and Prevention, provided the following definition (Bateman 2008): "Asthma is a chronic inflammatory disorder of the airways in which many cells and cellular elements play a role. The chronic inflammation is associated with airway hyper-responsiveness that leads to recurrent episodes of wheezing, breathlessness, chest tightness, and coughing, particularly at night or in the early morning. These events are usually associated with widespread, but variable, airflow obstruction within the lung that is often reversible either spontaneously or with treatment."

Q: What causes asthma?

A: The cause of asthma is not yet known. Through multiple studies, medical researchers have established that the disease is a special type of inflammation of the airway that leads to contraction of airway muscle, mucus production and swelling in the airways. The airways become overly responsive to environmental changes. The result is wheezing, coughing, and shortness of breath.

Q: Can asthma be cured?

A: At this time, there is no cure for asthma, but asthma can be controlled with the proper treatment. People with asthma can use medicines prescribed by their physicians to prevent or relieve their symptoms, and they can learn ways to manage their episodes better. They also can learn how to identify and avoid the things that trigger an episode. By educating themselves about medications and other asthma management strategies, most people with asthma can gain control of the disease and live an active life.

Q: Is asthma a psychological or emotional disease?

A: No. Although episodes of asthma can sometimes be brought on by strong emotions, it is important to know that asthma is not the result of emotional factors, such as a troubled parent-child relationship. Years ago, people more commonly believed that asthma was "all in one's head" and therefore not a real illness. Physicians and other medical researchers today know that this is incorrect.

Q: What are the most common asthma triggers?

A: Asthma is usually triggered by either common respiratory viruses, such as cold viruses, influenza viruses, parainfluenza viruses, respiratory syncytial viruses, or allergens, such as pollens from trees, grasses, weed, or mold, animal dander, dust mites, and cockroach particles.

Q: Is any method I can use to remove these asthma triggers?

A: Yes. You can use the AsthmaCare™ Kit to remove these asthma triggers from your upper airway.

Q: How is asthma diagnosed?

A: Asthma is sometimes hard to diagnose because it can resemble other respiratory problems such as emphysema, bronchitis and lower respiratory infections. For that reason, asthma is generally under-diagnosed. This means that many people with the disease do not know they have it and, therefore, do not receive treatment. Sometimes, the only symptom is a chronic cough, especially at night. On the other hand, coughing and/or wheezing may occur only with exercise. Some people mistakenly think they are having recurrent bronchitis, since respiratory infections usually settle in the chest of a person predisposed to asthma.

Q: How do I know if my symptoms are from asthma?

A: To diagnose asthma and distinguish it from other lung disorders, physicians rely on a combination of medical history, a thorough physical examination, and certain laboratory tests. These tests include spirometry (using an instrument that measure the air taken

10. Frequently Asked Questions about Asthma

into and out of the lungs), peak flow monitoring (another measure of lung function), chest X-rays and, sometimes, blood and allergy tests.

Q: What does an asthma attack feel like and what happens during an attack?

A: An asthma episode feels somewhat like taking deep breaths of very cold air on a winter day. Breathing becomes harder and may hurt, and there may be coughing. Breathing may make a wheezing or whistling sound. These problems occur because the airways of the lungs are getting narrower. The muscles that surround the airways tighten, the inner lining of the airways swells and pushes inward, and the membranes that line the airways secrete extra mucus, which can form plugs that further block the air passages. The rush of air through the narrowed airways produces the wheezing sounds that are typical of asthma.

Q: Are there support groups for people with asthma?

A: There are several asthma support groups. One national organization is the Allergy and Asthma Network's Mothers of Asthmatics (http://www.aanma.org/). Another is the -Asthma and Allergy Foundation of America (http://www.aafa.org/). There also is a Food Allergy and Anaphylaxis Network (http://www.foodallergy.org/).

Q: What is an allergy?

A: An allergy is an abnormal immune reaction against certain foreign or body-generated substances. The body automatically defends itself against harmful invaders such as viruses, bacteria, fungi or other microorganisms. However, in some people, the body overreacts to harmless substances, such as dust, mold or pollen, by producing a special antibody called immunoglobulin E (IgE). When patients with an allergic disease such as rhinitis are exposed to these substances, the immune system wrongly rallies its defenses, launching a host of complex chemical weapons to attack and destroy the supposed enemy. In the process, some destructive and, in extreme cases, life-threatening symptoms may be experienced.

Q: What causes an allergic reaction?

A: Allergens are ordinary substances can trigger allergic reactions. There are hundreds or even thousands of substances that can be an allergen. Among the most common are plant pollens, molds, household dust (dust mites), animal dander, industrial chemicals, foods (peanuts, wheat, dairy, etc.), medicines (penicillin, aspirin, etc.) and insect stings or bites.

Q: Where can an allergic reaction occur?

A: An allergic reaction may occur anywhere in the body, but usually appears on the skin, or in the eyes, lining of the stomach, nose, sinuses, throat and lungs; places where special immune system cells are already stationed to fight off any invaders that are inhaled, swallowed or come in contact with the skin.

Q: Who develops allergies?

A: Allergies can affect anyone, regardless of age, gender, race or socioeconomic status. While it is true that allergies are more common in children, they can occur for the first time at any age or, in some cases, recur after many years of remission.

Q: Are there genetic factors linked to allergies?

A: Although the exact genetic factors are not yet understood, the tendency to have allergies, or an allergic disease, is linked to heredity.

Q: What is the best method of testing for allergies?

A: The first step in diagnosing allergies is a thorough health history and physical examination. If you have allergy symptoms that occur in association with exposure to certain things, that is usually indicative of an allergy. Allergy diagnostic tests, such as skin tests or blood tests, provide similar information and merely confirm what your physician already knows from your health history.

10. Frequently Asked Questions about Asthma

Q: What if I don't know what factors are causing my allergies?

A: If you are unable to tell your doctor what could be the source of your allergies, your doctor will rely exclusively on the results of skin or blood tests. Because a health history is considered the most reliable tool in diagnosing allergies, relying solely on skin or blood tests could lead to a misdiagnosis of an allergic problem that you do not necessarily have.

Q: Under what circumstances would I need a skin test?

A: Skin tests, in most situations, are preferable because: (1) the results are available immediately; (2) they are less expensive than blood tests; and (3) they are more sensitive to subtle allergies.

Q: Under what circumstances would I need a blood test?

A: A blood test is appropriate in certain situations, particularly when you: (1) cannot suspend antihistamine therapy; (2) have a widespread skin disease; (3) are so sensitive to the allergen that the test might be risky; and (4) cannot be skin tested for some other reason.

Q: What are allergy shots?

A: Also known as immunotherapy, allergy shots are an effective and safe treatment for people who suffer from a variety of allergic diseases, including allergic rhinitis (hay fever), and insect stings. The treatment is also known as allergy immunization. Regardless of the name, the shots work by introducing small amounts of specially purified substances to which the person is allergic, in gradually increasing amounts. The allergy shots improve the patient's natural resistance to the allergens and minimize or eliminate the need for medications. After a successful immunotherapy, the patient will be no long allergic to that specific substance.

Q: Do allergy shots have side effects?

A: Like all medical treatments, allergy shots can have side effects. Your physician will discuss this with you in detail. Under no circumstances should you consider allergy shots without at least an attempt at avoidance of the troublesome allergen. For instance, cat allergy shots are no substitute for cat avoidance. Some allergens, though, such as grass pollen, are almost unavoidable and may require allergy shots to ease the symptoms of the allergic reaction.

Q: Why is it that frequent exposure to an allergen can increase sensitivity and cause allergic reaction, yet repeated exposure to an allergen in allergy shots helps build up immunity?

A: Regularly scheduled, repeated exposure to small amounts of an allergen can lead to immunity, whereas infrequent and erratic exposure to known or large amounts does not confer immunity; instead, it only increases the likelihood of producing allergen sensitization. Irregular exposure to allergens can lead to the production of allergy-specific IgE. The presence of these antibodies, when exposed to an allergen, can lead to an allergic reaction.

Q: Can IgE be changed with allergy shots?

A: Yes. During immunotherapy, allergen exposure is closely regulated and given on a scheduled basis. Small amounts of allergens are given over a period to build up to maintenance doses. This leads to the production of blocking antibodies (called IgG antibodies) and a decrease in the level of IgE-mediated antibodies.

Q: What is homeopathic therapy?

A: Homeopathy is based on utilizing progressively diluted infusions from plant, mineral and animal extracts. These are then produced in a liquid or tablet form with particular remedies prescribed for specific ailments or conditions. Their efficacy and potency are derived from this process of dilution, which is believed to leave the water or liquid with a memory of the extract. Homeopathy is also based on the principle of the body healing itself, aided by a remedy that mimics the symptom, or "like healing like". A homeopath (a special doctor who practices homeopathy) will typically assess all aspects of your lifestyle and health, and prescribe a remedy based on these factors, as well as your range of symptoms.

Q: What are the benefits of homeopathy?

A: The benefits of homeopathy include improved energy levels, individual attention, diagnosis and treatment, support for the

10. Frequently Asked Questions about Asthma

immune system; and a natural, holistic treatment without clinically noticeable side effects.

Q: How Can Homeopathy Help Asthma?

A: Homeopathy has a huge range of remedies for practically every ailment and illness, including asthma. To find out the best homeopathic medicines for your particular type of asthma, always consult a qualified and accredited homeopath that adheres to the professional conduct and standards of homeopathy. Also, if you use an over-the-counter (OTC) drug of homeopathy, remember that the more ingredients, the broader the protection.

Q: Why should I perform a nasal cleanse?

A: Everyone breathes every minute, of every hour, of every day. While breathing, everyone constantly inhales pollutants from the environment. If you do not cleanse them out, these pollutions will cause an inflammation, which often leads to a cold. Other times, you inhale viruses coughed or sneezed out by your family members or your co-workers. If you do not cleanse these viruses out, they will cause an infection within your nose.

Q: Why should I use the NasalCare® Nasal Cleanse Kit to do a nasal cleanse?

A: The NasalCare® Nasal Cleanse Kit has an award winning irrigator and premium solution. Using this system, you will have no risk to have the contaminated solution flows back into your sinuses.

Q: Why I should Use the AsthmaCare™ Kit to manage my asthma?

A: The AsthmaCare™ Kit provides you with an award winning nasal irrigator, premium nasal rinse packets, and a unique spray made with 23 active homeopathic ingredients. By using this kit, you can remove any inhaled asthma triggers, including viruses and allergens, thus reducing the oversensitivity of your airway during an asthma flare-up or attack. This kit is made with a patent-pending technology that no other manufacturer can supply.

Glossary

Acetaminophen: A pain reliever and fever reducer. Brand name: Tylenol®. The exact mechanism of action of acetaminophen is not known. Acetaminophen relieves pain by elevating the pain threshold (that is, by requiring a greater amount of pain to develop before it is felt by a person). Acetaminophen reduces fever through its action on the heat-regulating center (the "thermostat") of the brain. Generic is available.

Acquired: Anything that is not present at birth but develops some time later. In medicine, the word "acquired" implies "new" or "added."An acquired condition is "new" in the sense that it is not genetic (inherited) and "added" in the sense that was not present at birth.

Adenovirus: A group of viruses responsible for a spectrum of respiratory disease as well as infection of the stomach/intestine (gastroenteritis), eyes (conjunctivitis), and bladder (cystitis) and rash. Adenovirus respiratory diseases include a form of the Asthma, pneumonia, croup, and bronchitis. Patients with compromised immune systems are especially susceptible to severe complications of adenovirus infection. Acute respiratory disease (ARD), a disorder first recognized among military recruits during World War II, can be caused by adenovirus infections under conditions of crowding and stress.

Aloe vera: A short-stemmed plant with thick leaves with a soothing, viscous juice; leaves develop spiny margins with maturity; native to Mediterranean region; grown widely in tropics and as houseplants.

Antihistamines: Drugs that combat the histamine released during an allergic reaction by blocking the action of the histamine on the tissue. Since antihistamines do not stop the formation of histamine or the conflict between the antibody and antigen, they only protect tissues from some of the effects of an allergic reaction.

Antihistamines often cause mouth dryness and sleepiness. The "non-sedating" antihistamines may be less effective.

Asthma: A chronic respiratory disease, often arising from allergies that are characterized by sudden recurring attacks of labored breathing, chest constriction and coughing.

Bacteria: Single-celled microorganisms, which can exist either as independent (free-living) organisms or as parasites (dependent upon another organism for life).

Buffer: A buffer is a solution containing either a weak acid and its salt or a weak base and its salt, which is resistant to changes in pH.

Chest pain: There are many causes of chest pain. One is angina, which results from inadequate oxygen supply to the heart muscle. Angina can be caused by coronary artery disease or spasm of the coronary arteries. Chest pain can also be due to a heart attack (coronary occlusion) and other important diseases such as, for example, dissection of the aorta and a pulmonary embolism. Do not try to ignore chest pain and "work (or play) though it."Chest pain is a warning to seek medical attention.

Chills: Feelings of coldness accompanied by shivering. Chills may develop after exposure to a cold environment or may accompany a fever.

Chronic obstructive pulmonary disease (COPD): Any disorder that persistently obstructs bronchial airflow. COPD mainly involves two related diseases, chronic bronchitis and emphysema, which lead to the obstruction of airflow through the respiratory system. The condition is generally permanent and worsens over time.

Citric acid: A colorless translucent crystalline acid principally derived by fermentation of carbohydrates or from lemon, lime, and pineapple juices.

Conchae: Any turbinate bone, especially in the nose.

Turbinate: A bone in the nose that is situated along the sidewall of the nose and is covered by mucous membrane.

Common cold: A viral upper respiratory tract infection. Many different types of viruses can cause this contagious illness, and it is impossible for the body to build up resistance to all of them. This makes colds a frequent and recurring problem.

Congestion: An abnormal or excessive accumulation of a bodily fluid. Examples include nasal congestion (excess mucus and secretions in the air passages of the nose) seen with an Asthma and congestion of blood in the lower extremities seen with some types of heart failure.

Coronavirus: One of a group of viruses, which look like a corona (halo) when viewed under an electron microscope. This appearance is due to an array of surface projections.

Discharge: The flow of fluid from a part of the body, such as the nose.

Eustachian tube: The tube that runs from the middle ear to the nasopharynx. Eustachian tube protects, aerates and drains the middle ear. Blockage of the Eustachian tube leads to inflammation of the middle ear. The Eustachian tube is also called the otopharyngeal tube (because it connects the ear to the pharynx) and the auditory tube (and in Latin, the tuba acustica, tuba auditiva, and tuba auditoria).

Fatigue: A condition characterized by a reduced work capacity and efficiency of accomplishment, usually accompanied by tiredness. Fatigue can come on suddenly or be chronic and persist.

Flu: Short for influenza. Viruses that infect the respiratory tract cause the flu. Most people who get the flu recover completely in 1 to 2 weeks, but some people develop serious and potentially life-threatening medical complications, such as pneumonia. Much of the illness and death caused by influenza can be prevented by annual influenza vaccination.

Hoarseness: Hoarseness is a term referring to abnormal voice changes. Hoarseness may be manifested as a voice that sounds breathy, strained, rough, raspy, or a voice that has higher or lower pitch. There are many causes of hoarseness, including viral laryngitis, vocal cord nodules, laryngeal papillomas, gastroesophageal reflux-related laryngitis, and environmental irritants (such as tobacco smoking). An accumulation of fluid in the vocal cords associated with hoarseness has been termed Reinke's edema. Reinke's edema may occur because of cigarette smoking or voice abuse (prolonged or extended talking or shouting). Rarely, hoarseness results from serious conditions such as cancers of the head and neck region.

Ibuprofen: A non-steroidal anti-inflammatory drug (NSAID) commonly used to treat pain, swelling, and fever. Common brand names for Ibuprofen include Advil®, Motrin®, and Nuprin®.

Incubation period: In medicine, the time from initial exposure to an infectious agent till the appearance of the first signs and symptoms of the disease.

Isotonic: When a solution has the same osmotic pressure (concentration) as serum, which has a normal value of osmolality between 270–300 mOsm/kg water. Hypertonic: osmolality is higher than 300 mOsm/kg water; Hypotonic: osmolality is lower than 270 mOsm/kg water. See also "osmolality."

Mucus: A thick slippery fluid produced by the membranes lining certain organs such as the nose, mouth, throat, and vagina. Mucus is the Latin word for "a semi fluid, slimy discharge from the nose." Note that *mucus* is a noun while the adjective is *mucous*.

Nasal cavity: The vaulted chamber that lies between the floor of the cranium and the roof of the mouth of higher vertebrates extending from the external nares to the pharynx, being enclosed by bone or cartilage and usually incompletely divided into lateral halves by the septum of the nose, and having its walls lined with mucous membrane that is rich in venous plexuses and ciliated in the lower part which forms the beginning of the respiratory passage and warms and filters the inhaled air and that is modified as sensory epithelium in the upper olfactory part.

Nasal mucus: A slippery, sometimes thick, fluid produced by the membranes lining the nose. Excessive nasal mucus underlies a runny nose.

Onset: In medicine, the first appearance of the signs or symptoms of an illness. See also "incubation period."

Osmolality: The concentration of a solution in terms of osmoles of solutes per kilogram of solvent. Serum osmolality is a measure of the number of dissolved particles per unit of water in serum. The fewer the particles of solute in proportion to the number of units of water (solvent), the less concentrated the solution. Measurement of the serum osmolality indicates the hydration status within the cells because the osmotic equilibrium is constantly maintained on both sides of the cell membrane. Water moves freely back and forth across the membrane in response to the osmolar pressure being exerted by the molecules of solute in the intracellular and extracellular fluids. The normal value for serum osmolality is 270–300 mOsm/kg water. See also "isotonic."

Over-the-counter (OTC): A drug or a medical device that can be purchased by the consumer without a physician's prescription.

Parainfluenza: A disease due to an acute respiratory infection caused by a parainfluenza virus, usually occurring in children. It may present as anything from a relatively mild influenza-like illness to bronchitis, croup, and pneumonia.

Pathogenesis: The development of a disease. The origin of a disease and the chain of events leading to that disease.

Pulmonary: Having to do with the lungs.

Resistance: Opposition or the ability to withstand something. For example, some forms of staphylococcus are resistant to treatment with antibiotics.

Respiratory syncytial virus (RSV): A virus that causes mild respiratory infections, colds, and coughs in adults, but can produce severe respiratory problems, including bronchitis and pneumonia in young children. Patients with compromised immune, cardiac or pulmonary systems are at high risk.

Runny nose: Rhinorrhea is the medical term for this common problem. From the Greek words "rhinos" meaning "of the nose" and "rhoia" meaning, "a flowing."

Saline: Relating to salt. As an adjective, "saline" means, "containing salt." As a noun, "saline" is a salt solution, often adjusted to the normal salinity of the human body.

Sea salt: It is produced by the evaporation of seawater and that contains sodium chloride and trace elements such as sulfur, magnesium, zinc, potassium, calcium, and iron.

Secretion: A process in which a gland or tissue produces a biochemical and releases it for use by the organism or for excretion.

Sinus: An air-filled cavity in a dense portion of a skull bone. There are four pairs of sinuses: the frontal sinuses, behind the forehead; the maxillary sinuses, behind the cheeks; the sphenoid sinuses, behind the maxillary sinuses; and the ethmoid sinuses, behind the eyes. They are lined by mucous-secreting cells.

Sinusitis: Inflammation of the membrane lining the sinuses, which are directly connected to the nasal cavities.

Strep: Very commonly used shortened form of Streptococcus, a very common and important group of bacteria.

Strep throat: Strep throat is an infection caused by a type of bacteria called streptococcus, which can lead to serious complications if not adequately treated.

Syndrome: A set of signs and symptoms that tend to occur together and which reflect the presence of a particular disease or an increased chance of developing a particular disease.

TCID$_{50}$: The 50 percent viral tissue culture infectious dose; the level of viruses needed to cause an infection in half of the inoculated cells.

Vaccine: A preparation of a weakened or killed pathogen (bacterium or virus), or of a portion of the pathogen's structure that, when administered through injection or inhalation, stimulates antibody production or cellular immunity against the pathogen. Since the pathogen used is either weakened or killed, or just a portion of the full structure, it is incapable of causing severe infection, though it may cause side effects.

Virus: An infectious agent smaller than a bacterium, which cannot grow or reproduce apart from a living cell. A virus invades living cells and uses their chemical machinery to stay alive and to replicate itself.

Glossary

References

Abadie WM, McMains KC, and Weitzel EK. Irrigation penetration of nasal delivery systems: A cadaver study. Int Forum Allergy Rhinol, 2011; 1:46-49.

Adam P, Stiffman M, and Blake RL. A Clinical Trial of Hypertonic Saline Nasal Spray in Subjects With the Cold or Rhinosinusitis. Arch Fam Med. 1998;7:39-43.

Akinbami, LJ, Moorman JE, Bailey C. et al. Trends in Asthma Prevalence, Health Care Use, and Mortality in the United States, 2001–2010. NCHS Data Brief. No. 94. May 2012.

Alho OP, Karttunen R, and Karttunen TJ. Nasal mucosa in natural colds: effects of allergic rhinitis and susceptibility to recurrent sinusitis. Clin Exp Immu. 2004; 37 (2):366-72.

Anderson SD, Daviskas E, and Biomed ME. The mechanism of exercise-induced asthma is… J Allergy Clin Immunol 2000;106:453-459.

Ao HF, Wang Q, Jiang BF and He CY. Efficacy and Mechanism of Nasal Irrigation with a Hand Pump against Influenza and Non-Influenza Viral Upper Respiratory Tract Infection. Journal of Infectious Diseases and Immunity. 2011; Vol. 3(6):96-105.

Bachmann G, Hommel G, and Michel O: Effect of irrigation of the nose with isotonic salt solution on adult patients with chronic paranasal sinus disease. Eur Arch Otorhinolaryngol. 2000; 257(10): 537-41.

Baker DH. Iodine Toxicity and Its Amelioration. Exp Biol Med. 2004; 229:473–478.

Barrett BP, Brown RL, Locken K, et al. Treatment of the Asthma with unrefined echinacea: a randomized, double-blind, placebo-controlled trial. Annals of Internal Medicine. 2002;137(12):939–946.

Bateman ED, S. S. Hurd SS, P. J. Barnes PJ et al. Global strategy for asthma management and prevention: GINA executive summary. Eur Respir J. 2008 Jan;31(1):143-78.

Benninger MS. Nasal Mucociliary Transport after Exposure to Swimming Pool Water. American Journal of Rhinology, 1994; 8(5): 207-209.

Boston M, Dobratz EJ, Buescher ES, and Darrow DH. Effects of Nasal Saline Spray on Human Neutrophils. Arch Otolaryngol Head Neck Surg. 2003;129:660-664.

Brown CL, Graham SM. Nasal irrigations: good or bad? Curr Opin Otolaryngol Head Neck Surg, 2004; 12(1):9-13.

Butler CC, Robling M, Prout H, et al. Management of suspected acute viral upper respiratory tract infection in children with intranasal sodium cromoglicate: a randomised controlled trial. The Lancet 2002; 359 (9324): 2153-2158.

Casale TB, Romero FA, and Spierings EL. Intranasal noninhaled carbon dioxide for the symptomatic treatment of seasonal allergic rhinitis. J Allergy Clin Immunol. 2008; 121(1):105-109.

Cate TR, Couch RB, and Johnson KM. Studies with rhinovirus in volunteers: production of illness, effect of naturally acquired antibody, and demonstration of a protective effect not associated with serum antibody. J Clin Invest 1964; 43:56-67.

Cazacu AC, Greer J, Taherivand M and Demmler GJ. Comparison of Lateral-Flow Immunoassay and Enzyme Immunoassay with Viral Culture for Rapid Detection of Influenza Virus in Nasal Wash Specimens from Children. J Clin Microbiology. 2003; 41(5): 2132-2134.

Chang EHE, Wong K, Philpott K, and Javer A. Sinus Irrigation Bottles: A Potential Source of Infection? Rhinology World Program, April 15-19, 2009, Page 47, ABSTRACT NUMBER 1653.

Chen Y, Hamati E, Lee PK et al. Rhinovirus Induces Airway Epithelial Gene Expression through Double-Stranded RNA and IFN-Dependent Pathways. Am J Respir Cell Mol Biol. 2006; 34(2): 192–203.

Chilvers MA, McKean M, and Rutman A. et al. The effects of coronavirus on human nasal ciliated respiratory epithelium. Eur Respir J 2001; 18:965-970.

Couch RB. Rhinoviruses. In: Fields Virology, third edition, edited by B.N. Fields, D.M. Knipe, P.M. Howley, et al. Lippincott –Raven Publishers, Philadelphia 1996; Chapter 23, pp.713-734.

Couch RB. The Asthma: Control. J Infect Dis 1984, 150: 167-73.

Douglas RG Jr, Cate TR, Gerone JP, Couch RB. Quantitative rhinovirus shedding patterns in volunteers. Am Rev Respir Dis. 1966; 94:159-167.

Eby GA, Davis DR, and Halcomb WW. Reduction in duration of Asthma by zinc gluconate lozenges in a double-blind study. Antimicrobial Agents Chemotherapy 1984; 25:20-4.

Eby GA. Zinc lozenges as cure for the Asthma – A review and hypothesis. Medical Hypotheses 2010; 74: 482–492.

Eccles R. Understanding the symptoms of the Asthma and influenza. Lancet Infect Dis 2005;5: 718–725.

Falsey AR, Formica MA, Treanor JJ and Walsh EE. Comparison of Quantitative Reverse Transcription-PCR to Viral Culture for Assessment of Respiratory Syncytial Virus Shedding. J Clin Microbiology. 2003; 41(9): 4160–4165.

Feily A, Namazi MR. Aloe vera in dermatology: a brief review. G Ital Dermatol Venereol. 2009; 144(1):85-91.

Fendrick AM, Monto AS, Nitghtengale B and Sanes M. The Economic Burdon of Non-Influenza-Related Viral Respiratory Tract Infection in the United States. Arch Intern Med. 2003: 163:487-494.

Folkerts G, Busse WW, Nijkamp FP, Sorkness R, and Gern JE. Virus-induced Airway Hyperresponsiveness and Asthma. Am J Respir Crit Care Med 1998, Vol 157. pp 1708–1720.

Georgitis JW. Nasal hyperthermia and simple irrigation for perennial rhinitis. Changes in inflammatory mediators. Chest, 1994; 106:1487-92.

Gern GE, Mosser AG, and Swenson CA. Inhibition of Rhinovirus Replication In Vitro and In Vivo by Acid-Buffered Saline. The Journal of Infectious Diseases 2007; 195:1137–1143.

Gern JE, Dick EC, Lee WW, and Murray S. Rhinovirus enters but does not replicate inside monocytes and airway macrophages. J. Immunology, 1996; 156(2): 621-627.

Gern JE, Vrtis R, Grindle KA, Swenson C, and Busse WW. Relationship of upper and lower airway cytokines to outcome of experimental rhinovirus infection. Am J Respir Crit Care Med 2000;162:2226–2231.

Godfrey JC, Sloane B, Smith DS, et al. Zinc gluconate and the Asthma: A controlled clinical study. J Int Med Res 1992;20:234-46.

Griego SD, Weston CB, Adams JL. et al. Role of p38 Mitogen-Activated Protein Kinase in Rhinovirus-Induced Cytokine Production by Bronchial Epithelial Cells. The Journal of Immunology. 2000; 165: 5211–5220.

Gwaltney JM and Ruckert RR. Rhinovirus. In: Richmann DD, Whitley RJ, Hayden FG, eds. Clinical Virology. NY: Churchill Livingstone, 1997:1025-1047.

Gwaltney JM Jr. The Asthma. In: Mandell GL, Bennett JE, Dolin R, eds. Mandell, Douglas and Bennett's Principles and Practice of

Infectious Diseases. 4thed. New York: Churchill Livingstone, 1995:561-566.

Gwaltney JM, Hendley JO, Simon G, and Jordon WS. Rhinovirus infections in an industrial population. I. The occurrence of illness.. N Engl J Med 1966;275:1261-1268.

Hall CB and Douglas RJ. Clinically useful method for the isolation of respiratory syncytial virus, Journal of Infectious Diseases, 1975; 131: 1-5.

Hall CB and ouglas, R.J. Quantitative shedding patterns of respiratory syncytial virus in infants, Journal of Infectious Diseases, 1975; 132: 151-156.

Hall CB, Geiman JM, Breese BB, and Douglas RJ: Parainfluenza virus infections in children: Correlation of shedding with clinical manifestations, *Journal of Pediatrics*, 1977; 91: 194-198.

Harkema J, Carey S, and Wagner JG. The Nose Revisited: A Brief Review of the Comparative Structure, Function, and Toxicological Pathology of the Nasal Epithelium. Toxicological Pathology, 2006; 34:252–269.

Hashimoto S and Bel EH. Targeting IL-5 in severe asthma: a DREAM come true? The Lancet 2012, Vol 380 (9842) August 18–24, 626.

Hauptman G and Ryan MW. The effect of saline solutions on nasal patency and mucociliary clearance in rhinosinusitis patients. Otolaryngol Head Neck Surg. 2007; 137(5):815-21.

Heatley DG, McConnell KE, Kille TL, Leverson GE. Nasal irrigation for the alleviation of sinonasal symptoms, Otolaryngol Head Neck Surg. 2001;125(1):44-48.

Hemila H. Vitamin C and the Asthma. British Journal of Nutrition. 1992; 61, 3-16.

Holgate ST, Davies DE, Puddicombe S. et al. Mechanisms of airway epithelial damage: epithelial-mesenchymal interactions in the pathogenesis of asthma. Eur Respir J 2003; 22(Suppl. 44): 24s–29s.

Jackson GG and Muldoon RL. Viruses causing common respiratory infection in man. I. Rhinoviruses. J Infect Dis 1973; 127:328-355.

Jackson JL, Lesho E, and Peterson C. Zinc and the Asthma: A meta-analysis revisited. J Nutr 2000; 130(5S Suppl):1512S-1015S.

Jakiela B, Brockman-Schneider R and Amineva S et al. Basal Cells of Differentiated Bronchial Epithelium Are More Susceptible to Rhinovirus Infection. Am J Respir Cell Mol Biol 2008; 38: 517–523.

Johnston SL, Papi A, Bates PJ et al. Low Grade Rhinovirus Infection Induces a Prolonged Release of IL-8 in Pulmonary Epithelium. The Journal of Immunology. 1998; 160: 6172–6181.

Johnston SL. Overview of Virus-induced Airway Disease. The Proceedings of the American Thoracic Society 2005; 2:150-156.

Kaliner M. Treatment of Sinusitis in the Next Millennium. Allergy & Asthma Proceedings. 1998;19:181.

Kaul P, Biagioli MC and Singh I. Rhinovirus-Induced Oxidative Stress and Interleukin-8 Elaboration Involves p47-phox but Is Independent of Attachment to Intercellular Adhesion Molecule-1 and Viral Replication. The Journal of Infectious Diseases 2000;181:1885-1890.

Kaul P, Singh I and Turner RB. Effect of Nitric Oxide on Rhinovirus Replication and Virus-Induced Interleukin-8 Elaboration. AM J RESPIR CRIT CARE MED 1999;159:1193-1198.

Kopf M, Bachmann, MF; Marsland, BJ. Averting inflammation by targeting the cytokine environment. Nature Reviews Drug Discovery. 2010, 9(9):703-18.

Korant BD and Butterworth BE. Inhibition by zinc of rhinovirus protein cleavage: Interaction of zinc with capsid polypeptides. J Virol 1976; 18:298-306.

Korant BD, Kauer JC, and Butterworth BE. Zinc ions inhibit replication of rhinoviruses. Nature 1974; 248:588-590.

Lavigne F, Tulic MK, Gagnon J, and Hamid Q. Selective irrigation of the sinuses in the management of chronic rhinosinusitis refractory to medical therapy: a promising start. J Otolaryngol-Head Neck Surg. 2004; 33(1):10-16.

Lee N, Chan PKS, Hui DSC et al. Viral Loads and Duration of Viral Shedding in Adult Patients Hospitalized with Influenza. The Journal of Infectious Diseases 2009; 200:492-500.

Liu J. and Zhang L. A unique device to deliver the cleanse liquid to nasal and sinus cavities. China Patent granted on October 11, 2006, Patent Number ZL200520086805.9.

Liu J. and Zhang L. The unique solutions for nasal irrigation. China Patent granted on February 14, 2007, Patent Number ZL2004 10024220.4.

Liu J. Nasal-nasopharyngeal cleaning system. US Patent 6238377, Issued on May 29, 2001.

Liu J. Nasal-nasopharyngeal cleaning system. US Patent 6736792, Issued on May 18, 2004.

Livingston E, Thomson NC, & Chalmers GW. Impact of Smoking on Asthma Therapy: A Critical Review of Clinical Evidence. Drugs, 2005, Volume 65, Number 11, pp. 1521-1536(16).

Manning SC: Pediatric Sinusitis. Otolaryngologic Clinics of North America. 1993; 26,4:623-637.

Meltzer EO, Hamilos DL, Hadley JA et al. Rhinosinusitis: Developing guidance for clinical trials. J. Allergy and Clinical Immunology 2006; 118(5): S17-S61.

Message SD and Johnston SL. Host defense function of the airway epithelium in health and disease: clinical background. J of Leukocyte Biology. 2004; 75(1): 5-17.

Michel O. Nasal irrigation in case of rhinosinusitis. Laryngorhinootologie. 2006; 85(6):448-58.

Mossad SB, Macknin ML, Medendorp SV, and Mason P. Zinc gluconate lozenges for treating the Asthma. A randomized, double-blind, placebo-controlled study. Ann Intern Med 1996; 125:81-88.

Murray CS, Simpson A, and Custovic A. Allergens, Viruses, and Asthma Exacerbations. Proc Am Thorac Soc 2004; vol 1. pp 99–104.

Nsouli TM, et al. Long-term use of nasal saline irrigation: Harmful or helpful? ACAAI, 2009; Abstract O32.

Olson DE, Rasgon BM, and Hilsinger RL. Radiographic comparison of three methods for nasal saline irrigation. Laryngoscope 2002; 112:1394–1398.

Panagiotopoulos G, Naxakis S, Papavasilious A, et al. Decreasing Nasal Mucus Ca+++ Improves Hyposmia. Rhinology. 2005; 43(2):130-134.

Papsin B and McTavish A. Saline nasal irrigation. Can Family Physician. 2003; 49:168-173.

Pavord ID, Korn S, Howarth P, Bleecker ER et al. Mepolizumab for severe eosinophilic asthma (DREAM): a multicentre, double-blind, placebo-controlled trial. The Lancet 2012, Vol 380 (9842) August 18–24, 651-659.

Pitkaranta A, Arruda E, Malmberg H, and Hayden FG. Detection of Rhinovirus in Sinus Brushings of Patients with Acute Community-Acquired Sinusitis by Reverse Transcription-PCR. J. Clin Microbiology 1997; 35: 1791–93.

Pynnonen MA, Mukerji SS, Kim HM, Adams ME, and Terrell JE. Nasal Saline for Chronic Sinonasal Symptoms, A Randomized Controlled Trial. Arch Otolaryngol Head Neck Surg. 2007; 133(11):1115-1120.

Rabago D et al. Efficacy of daily saline nasal irrigation among patients with sinusitis: a randomized controlled trial. J Family Practice. 2003; 51(12): 1049-55.

Rabago D, Barrett B, Marchand L, Maberry R, and Mundt M. Qualitative Aspects of Nasal Irrigation Use by Patients With Chronic Sinus Disease in a Multimethod Study Annals of Family Medicine 2006; 4:295-301.

Rabago D, et al. The efficacy of hypertonic saline nasal irrigation for chronic sinonasal symptoms. Otolaryngol Head Neck Surg. 2005; 133(1):3-8.

Rabago D, Guerard E, Bukstein D. Nasal irrigation for chronic sinus symptoms in patients with allergic rhinitis, asthma, and nasal polyposis.WMJ. 2008; 107(2):69-75.

Rabone SJ and Saraswati SB: Acceptance and effects of nasal lavage in volunteer woodworkers. Occup Med (Lond), 1999; 49:365-369.

Rachelevsky GS, Slavin RG, and Wald ER. Sinusitis: Acute, Chronic and Manageable. Patient Care. 1997; 131:4.

Ravizza R and Fornadley J. Irrigation of the Nose Helps Prevent Colds. The 50th Scientific Assembly of the American Academy of Family Physicians. San Francisco, Sept 21, 1998.

Rider TH, Zook CE, Boettcher TL, Wick ST, and Pancoast JS et al. Broad-Spectrum Antiviral Therapeutics. PLoS ONE 2011; 6(7): e22572. doi:10.1371/.

Scheid DC and Hamm RM. Acute bacterial rhinosinusitis in adults: part II. Treatment. Am Fam Physician. 2004; 70(9):1642, 1645.

Scott C. Pediatric sinusitis, Manning. In: Inflammatory Diseases of the Sinuses. Otolaryngologic Clinics of North America. 1993; 26:623-638.

Scott EJ and Heath GF. Factors Affecting the Growth of Rhinovirus 2 in Suspension Cultures of L 132 Cells. J. Gen. Virology 1970; 6:5-24.

Sehra S, Pynaert G, Tournoy K, Haegeman A, Matthys P, Tagawa Y, Pauwels R, Grooten J. Airway IgG counteracts specific and bystander allergen-triggered pulmonary inflammation by a mechanism dependent on Fc gamma R and IFN-gamma . J Immunol. 2003 Aug 15;171(4):2080-9.

Shah SA, Sander CS and White CM. Evaluation of echinacea for the prevention and treatment of the Asthma: a meta-analysis. The Lancet Infectious Diseases. 2007; 7(7): 473-480.

Shoseyov D, et al. Treatment with hypertonic saline versus normal saline nasal wash of pediatric chronic sinusitis. J Allergy Clin Immunol. 1998; 101(5): 602-605.

Slapak I, Skoupá J, Strnad P, and Horník P. Efficacy of isotonic nasal wash (seawater) in the treatment and prevention of rhinitis in children. Arch Otolaryngol Head Neck Surg. 2008; 134(1):67-74.

Statistics Canada, Asthme, 2010. Website http://www.statcan.gc.ca/pub/82-625-x/2011001/article/11458-eng.htm

Talbot AR, Herr MH, and Parsons DS. Mucociliary clearance and buffered hypertonic saline solution. Laryngoscope 1997; 107:500-503.

Tano L and Tano K. A Daily Nasal Spray with Saline Prevents Symptoms of Rhinitis. Acta Oto-laryngologica, 2004; 124(9):1059-1062.

Taylor JA, Weber W, and Standish L. Efficacy and Safety of Echinacea in Treating Upper Respiratory Tract Infections in Children. JAMA. 2003;290(21):2824-2830.

Tomooka, LT, Murphy C, and Davidson TM. Clinical Study and Literature Review of Nasal Irrigation. The Laryngoscope. 2000; 110(7):1189–1193.

Tsao CH, Chen LC, Yeh KW and Huang JL. Concomitant Chronic Sinusitis Treatment in Children With Mild Asthma. The Effect on Bronchial Hyper-responsiveness. CHEST 2003; 123:757–764.

Turetsky BT, Glass CA, Abbazia J. et al. Reduced Posterior Nasal Cavity Volume: A Gender-Specific Neuro-developmental Abnormality in Schizophrenia. Schizophr Res. 2007; 93(1-3): 237–244.

Turner RB, Bauer R, Woelkart K, Hulsey TC et al. An Evaluation of Echinacea angustifolia in Experimental Rhinovirus Infections. N Engl J Med 2005; 353:341-348.

Wark PAB, Johnston SL, Moric I, Simpson JL Hensley MJ, & Gibson PG. Neutrophil degranulation and cell lysis is associated with clinical severity in virus-induced asthma. Eur Respir J 2002; 19: 68–75.

Wedzicha JA and Donaldson GC. Exacerbations of Chronic Obstructive Pulmonary Disease. RESPIRATORY CARE. 2003; 48(12):1204-1213.

Welch KC, Cohen MB, Doghramji LL. et al. Clinical correlation between irrigation bottle contamination and clinical outcomes in post-functional endoscopic sinus surgery patients. Am J Rhinol Allergy 2009; 23, 401–404.

Wilkinson TMA, Hurst JR, Perera WR et Al. Effect of Interactions between Lower Airway Bacterial and Rhinoviral Infection in Exacerbations of COPD. CHEST 2006; 129:317–324.

Wormald PJ, Cain T, Oates L, Hawke L, and Wong I. A comparative study of three methods of nasal irrigation. Laryngoscope, 2004; 114:2224-2227.

Yu H, Dong Z, and Yang Z. Molecular biological study of aloe vera in the treatment of experimental allergic rhinitis in rat. Lin Chuang Er Bi Yan Hou Ke Za Zhi. 2002; 16(5):229-31.

Zeiger RS and Schatz M. Chronic Rhinitis: A Practical Approach to Diagnosis and Treatment. Immunology & Allergy Practice. 1982; 4(4):26-35.

Zeiger RS. Prospects for ancillary treatment of rhinosinusitis in the 1990's. J Allergy Clin Immunol. 1992; 90:478.

Zhu L, Lee PK, Lee WM et al. Rhinovirus-Induced Major Airway Mucin Production Involves a Novel TLR3-EGFR–Dependent Pathway. Am J Respir Cell Mol Biol 2009; 40: 610–619.

About the Author

Dr. James Z. Liu is a trained physician specializing in prevention and epidemiology of infectious diseases in Shandong University School of Preventive Medicine, and a doctor of philosophy (PhD) in Human Nutrition at the Pennsylvania State University. He has been a medical research scientist for thirty years with both academic institutions and pharmaceutical companies. During his early academic career, Dr. Liu published thirty-two peer-reviewed medical research articles and received numerous medical research awards from the central government, national professional societies, and academia.

While working for the pharmaceutical industry, Dr. Liu authored twelve US patents, and created and developed a number of new healthcare products. He has led multiple functional teams to conduct clinical trials for a number of top pharmaceutical companies during the last seventeen years. Currently at TechWorld Medicals, Dr. Liu continues his innovations and transforms medical sciences into practical technologies, and plays instrumental roles for gaining products approval/registration in US FDA and China SFDA.

The clinical study published in 2011 verified what Dr. Liu originally hypothesized when he filed the U.S. patent application in 1997: physically removing viruses from nasal and nasopharyngeal cavities can be an effective method to treat and prevent infectious diseases, like the Asthma. This book will help everyone on how to treat asthma safely, quickly and economically.

Dr. Liu has realized that many asthma triggers can be safely removed by using what he invented for curing the common cold. If these cold viruses, pollens, animal dander, air pollution are removed, these patients with asthma should have a decreased chance of having an asthma attack. In the past, many patients with asthma used Dr. Liu's invented nasal cleanse system and have experienced less frequent asthma attacks. Therefore, this book is written from the hypotheses behind the development and effectiveness of the nasal cleanse system as well as from actual user experience. Dr. Liu led his R&D team to develop this unique OTC product, AsthmaCare™ Kit, for these patients with asthma to gain freedom from asthma.

Dr. Liu is the author of the books "How to Cure a Cold in Two Days", "How We Cured Our Colds in One Day". Now Dr. Liu authors this book "You Too Can Be Free from Asthma" with a hope to help you to have a happy daily life.

About the Author

Made in the USA
Las Vegas, NV
06 July 2022